THE VITAMIN CURE

FOR

Chronic Fatigue Syndrome

JONATHAN E. PROUSKY, M.SC., N.D.

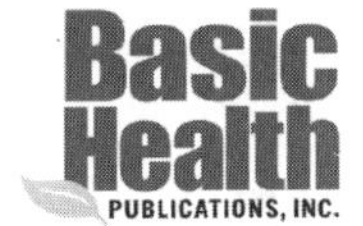

The information contained in this book is based upon the research and personal and professional experiences of the authors. It is not intended as a substitute for consulting with your physician or other healthcare provider. Any attempt to diagnose and treat an illness should be done under the direction of a healthcare professional.

The publisher does not advocate the use of any particular healthcare protocol but believes the information in this book should be available to the public. The publisher and authors are not responsible for any adverse effects or consequences resulting from the use of the suggestions, preparations, or procedures discussed in this book. Should the reader have any questions concerning the appropriateness of any procedures or preparation mentioned, the authors and the publisher strongly suggest consulting a professional healthcare advisor.

Basic Health Publications, Inc.
28812 Top of the World Drive
Laguna Beach, CA 92651
949-715-7327 • www.basichealthpub.com

Library of Congress Cataloging-in-Publication Data

Library of Congress Cataloging-in-Publication Data is available through the Library of Congress.

ISBN: 978-1-59120-268-4

Editor: John Anderson
Typesetting/Book design: Gary A. Rosenberg
Cover design: Mike Stromberg

Printed in the United States of America

10 9 8 7 6 5 4 3 2 1

CONTENTS

ACKNOWLEDGMENTS

I would like to thank Andrew Saul and Norman Goldfind of Basic Health Publications for giving me this opportunity and for including me in The Vitamin Cure series of books.

I thank my wife, Robin, for all that she does. She is the best and most capable person that I know, and above all, she is the love of my life. I am also indebted to my mother for her unconditional love and her all-around positive nature and zest for life.

To my brother, Brian, I am eternally grateful for your constant encouragement and genuine praise about my career, and for simply being such a great guy. To my father, you are a tremendous example of strength and fortitude, and know firsthand the experience of living with unrelenting fatigue and muscle weakness. Thank you for being such a generous and loving person.

FOREWORD

Chronic fatigue syndrome (CFS) and fibromyalgia represent an energy crisis in our bodies. In fact, they are illnesses of modern life caused by multiple problems, including poor nutrition, poor sleep, hormonal deficiencies, and other stresses (infections, injuries, toxic chemicals, and toxic bosses/spouses). Simply put, anything that causes you to spend more energy than you are able to create will result in an energy crisis. When this occurs, the area using the most energy for its size (the hypothalamus gland) malfunctions first, like blowing a fuse. This center controls sleep, hormones, temperature, and blood flow/blood pressure/sweating, and its malfunctioning causes many of the symptoms of CFS. In addition, if your muscles do not have enough energy, they will get stuck in the shortened position and you'll be in pain (think rigor mortis), which is then called fibromyalgia. The chronic pain then causes changes in your brain that amplifies the pain (central sensitization). CFS and its painful cousin fibromyalgia are increasing in epidemic proportions—by 400 to 1,000 percent in the last decade alone.

As Professor Prousky notes in this excellent book, chronic fatigue and fibromyalgia are *very* treatable. It is refreshing to see this well-thought-out and scientifically referenced overview of the importance of optimized nutritional support in CFS. It is especially important that it is written by not only a naturopath (who tend to be much more familiar with proper use of nutritional support than medical doctors) but one who is a professor of clinical nutrition at a school of naturopathy.

The book provides a broad foundation to help readers understand the diverse components factoring into chronic fatigue:

- A discussion of proper diagnosis
- Contributing factors, including environmental issues (toxins and infections), lifestyle and other factors, and nutrition
- An overview of how CFS impacts multiple body systems (such as blood cell fluidity, autonomic function, and so on)

This helps the reader to finally figure out why they have been feeling so poorly. In chronic fatigue, knowledge and understanding can be a critical first step in the healing process.

Professor Prousky also discusses the many important areas needing to be treated. These include mind-body issues, the importance of sleep, treating allergies (especially to foods), and much more. He recognizes that a comprehensive approach offers the best opportunity for cure. He also wisely advises that including psycho-spiritual issues as well as physical treatment is critical. As I often advise physicians, "If you get the patient well so they can return to a life they hate, you've done nothing for them!"

The good news, however, is that this is all very treatable. Nutritional and herbal support can be used to improve hormonal function. Many studies have shown immune system dysfunction in chronic fatigue and fibromyalgia, which can result in viral infections, bowel infections, and fungal/*Candida* infections. The nutritional therapies discussed in this book are helpful in supporting the immune system to eliminate infections.

The Vitamin Cure for Chronic Fatigue Syndrome is an excellent and powerful tool that will empower you to begin your own healing process. Everyone is different, and although this book can tell you which nutrients are most likely to help, individual needs vary considerably. Therefore, in applying Professor Prousky's guidance, check in with your body to see how the treatments make you feel. Keep doing the ones that leave you feeling better, and feel free to discard the others.

The comprehensive metabolic approach to treatment detailed in this book has proven to by highly effective for those suffering from chronic fatigue and fibromyalgia. Although focusing on nutritional support, this book gives you other powerful information for healing: on treating allergies, on restoring a healthy balance to bowel bacteria, and on detoxification. These are areas where naturopathy shines, and this book offers important guidance. Nutrition is a critical part of treatment, as it supports your body in healing itself. This will give you all the tools you need to get well, and *The Vitamin Cure for Chronic Fatigue Syndrome* will help you. Best wishes in your healing!

—Jacob E. Teitelbaum, M.D.

Dr. Teitelbaum is an international expert on chronic fatigue syndrome and the author of *From Fatigued to Fantastic!* and *Pain Free 1-2-3*.

INTRODUCTION

Imagine having such unrelenting and disabling fatigue that it is virtually impossible to do housework. I have heard people with chronic fatigue syndrome (CFS) recount stories in which daily tasks, such as cleaning, doing laundry, and even venturing to the corner store, became insurmountable. Now imagine that effective, natural, restorative treatments are prescribed. After some period of time, the person no longer feels as burdened by his or her unrelenting fatigue and is now living life more fully. I have personally witnessed tremendous quality-of-life improvements among CFS patients from the nutritional and other natural treatments described in this book.

Chronic fatigue is a syndrome in which the entire human organism has gone awry and is out of kilter. Because virtually every physiological system is affected by CFS, mainstream medical treatments attempt to treat it by utilizing several medications to specifically target the various features of the illness. For example, allopathic medicine often uses medications that increase a brain chemical known as serotonin in order to treat CFS-associated depression. Allopathic medical approaches also involve the use of analgesics, anticonvulsants, muscle relaxants, sleep medications, stimulants, and a host of other drugs to target specific problems encountered with chronic fatigue. This approach, while sometimes very helpful, can also be associated with many unwanted side effects and even increased morbidity. My clinical experiences with CFS patients have shown that they typically prefer a more natural approach because the treatments are more tolerable and the side effects are much less.

This is the first book on chronic fatigue, to my knowledge, that addresses the myriad of causes and systematically covers the restorative vitamin and other treatments capable of reducing CFS symptoms, helping the body to achieve more balance, and increasing quality of life. Vitamin treatments encompass many commonly used over-the-counter vitamins, such as vitamins B_1 (thiamine), B_2 (riboflavin), B_3 (niacin or niacinamide), C (ascorbic acid), and E (D-alpha tocopherol). Other treatments include minerals, such as magnesium and zinc, and herbal treatments, such as extracts of *Ginkgo biloba* and periwinkle (vinpocetine). I do not believe that consuming dietary sources of the nutrients that I recommend will have sufficient therapeutic value. I have purposely omitted recommending dietary sources of various nutrients because this book is not about eating specific foods rich in micronutrients (although I certainly advocate this) as a way to overcome chronic fatigue. Taking therapeutic doses of specific nutrients and other natural health products is the best way to effectively treat the debilitating symptoms that characterize CFS.

Chronic fatigue syndrome is considered by most authorities to be a difficult-to-treat and elusive medical condition. However, there is much hope and optimism now because treatments are available to make it a manageable chronic illness, allowing patients to live a more productive life with fewer flare-ups and exacerbations. Even though the natural treatments described in this book do not guarantee a cure for CFS, they do afford the most important ideal in medicine, which is to improve the lives of suffering patients.

Those with chronic fatigue should seriously and critically consider the treatment recommendations in this book. The majority of them can be safely used and combined with mainstream medical treatments, or they can be used as an alternative to orthodox treatments. Effective medical management and treatment is best done when supervised by a properly regulated (licensed) clinician.

These treatments can successfully improve the lives of those with chronic fatigue syndrome, and even the lives of patients with related medical conditions, such as fibromyalgia and multiple chemical sensitivity disorder. They are based on sound medical and scientific evidence, ranging from anecdotal case reports to clinical trials evaluating specific natural treatments. More than one treatment is usually recommended so as to facilitate better integration and healing among the many complex physiological systems affected by CFS, such as the central nervous system, the immune system, and the muscular system.

I hope that those of you with chronic fatigue will benefit from these complementary and alternative treatment options and find greater happiness and fulfillment in your life.

A Note to the Reader

- If you have not been diagnosed with chronic fatigue syndrome, please thoroughly read this book and pay particular attention to Chapter 1, which outlines precisely how CFS is diagnosed. To receive a proper diagnosis, it is best to see a licensed clinician, such as a naturopathic doctor, a chiropractor, a medical doctor, or an osteopathic physician.

- If you are taking any prescription or over-the-counter supplements or medications, you must consult with a licensed clinician before using any of the treatment options in this book.

- If you decide to utilize the vitamin and non-vitamin treatments as described in this book, please consult with a clinician experienced in natural medicine for further guidance and instruction. If your health-care provider is not experienced in this area, consider bringing this book with you to your appointment, as the recommendations are largely based on published studies in medical and scientific journals, which may prove useful in informing your doctor.

- For optimal results, all of these treatments should be used in conjunction with a comprehensive holistic treatment plan, which includes lifestyle and dietary modifications.

CHAPTER 1

WHAT IS CHRONIC FATIGUE SYNDROME?

In the autumn of 1984, in Incline Village, Nevada, local physicians Paul Cheney and Daniel Peterson documented the first cluster of approximately 200 people who became ill with a prolonged flu-like illness. They were perplexed because all of their patients had similar unexplained symptoms, including high levels of Epstein-Barr virus antibodies in their blood. This mysterious syndrome was referred to as chronic Epstein-Barr virus (CEBV). About a year later, a second cluster of similar flu-like symptoms appeared in Lyndonville, New York, but this time it primarily affected children and adolescents. The media became interested in these phenomena, and soon after there were sporadic reports of similar flu-like illnesses across the United States.[1]

Sometime during the 1980s, CEBV was nicknamed the "yuppie flu" because it was believed to primarily affect affluent, young professionals. This is completely untrue since the majority of people having the illness are between forty and fifty-nine years of age and are mostly lower-income as opposed to high-income earners. Eventually, the U.S. Centers for Disease Control and Prevention (CDC) became involved and named the illness chronic fatigue syndrome (CFS), and they also created a U.S. case definition for diagnosis in 1988.[2]

We know that CFS can suddenly arise after a bout of flu or other types of viral illnesses or even from a traumatic event like a motor vehicle accident. The majority of cases, however, manifest slowly and insidiously after many years of suffering from unrelenting and debilitating fatigue. In their book *Sick and Tired of Feeling Sick and Tired,* Paul J. Donoghue, Ph.D., and Mary E. Siegel, Ph.D., describe this type of fatigue: "The fatigue is relentless. Overexercise or overwork does not cause it and bed rest frequently fails to relieve it. It appears regardless of activity or inactivity, happiness or sadness. It simply exists in and of itself, and no medication, positive thought, or rest can relieve it."[3]

Fatigue is not the only problem that people with CFS experience. They often present with sleep difficulties, problems with concentration and short-term memory, flu-like symptoms, pain in the joints and muscles, tender lymph nodes, sore throat and headaches.

Chronic fatigue syndrome is not easy to diagnose: approximately 1 million Americans have it, yet less than 20 percent have actually received a proper diagnosis.[4] This low rate of diagnosis presents an urgent need for a better understanding of CFS, both by those suffering from it and by clinicians and other health-care professionals faced with patients manifesting these complex signs and symptoms.

Chronic fatigue affects 3–5 times more women than men and occurs in all ethnic and racial groups around the world. Prevalence rates internationally are as follows[5]:

- Japan: 0.85–1,500 cases per 100,000
- Australia: 37.1–1,500 cases per 100,000
- Netherlands: 112 cases per 100,000
- New Zealand: 127 cases per 100,000
- Brazil: 2,000 cases per 100,000
- Great Britain: 6–2,600 cases per 100,000
- Iceland: 1,400 cases per 100,000
- Italy: 9,500 cases per 100,000

Since the 1980s, when the first clusters were reported, to the present time, there have been numerous reports and publications validating the existence of CFS (sometimes referred to as chronic fatigue and immune dysfunction syndrome or CFIDS). While it is considered a legitimate medical illness by many knowledgeable clinicians and health-care professionals, there continues to be an aura of shame, stigma, and confusion associated with chronic fatigue. Even expert clinicians can find it difficult to diagnose, which merely leads to further frustration and the likely prescribing of ineffectual treatments to the unfortunate people who have it.

Because CFS is so complex, it cannot be diagnosed and treated in the same way as other medical conditions. To sort through the confusion, this chapter will highlight what fatigue is, how fatigue is different than CFS, how chronic fatigue is diagnosed, and the numerous factors implicated in causing this illness.

Diagnosing Chronic Fatigue

Being fatigued is a very unpleasant feeling. All of us have experienced temporary fatigue during the course of our lives, often as a result of eating the wrong diet, not sleeping well, staying up too late, having relationship conflicts, cramming for school exams, or dealing with an infection like the flu. When fatigue lasts longer than it should, medical attention is usually sought after. In these situations, a thorough medical evaluation is needed to determine if fatigue is due to an underlying medical reason.

COMMON UNDERLYING MEDICAL REASONS FOR FATIGUE[6]

SYSTEM INVOLVED	CAUSE
Cardiorespiratory	Heart disease, congestive heart failure, chronic obstructive pulmonary disease
Neuroendocrine	Hypothyroidism, hyperthyroidism, Addison's disease, Cushing's disease, diabetes
Gastrointestinal	Malignant disease, celiac disease, chronic liver disease, primary biliary cirrhosis

SYSTEM INVOLVED	CAUSE
Hematologic	Anemia, autoimmune disease, iron deficiency, lymphoma, leukemia
Infectious	Chronic Epstein-Barr virus, influenza, human immunodeficiency virus, other viral illnesses, tuberculosis, Lyme disease
Neuropsychiatric	Obstructive sleep syndromes (e.g., sleep apnea), multiple sclerosis, myasthenia gravis, Parkinson's disease, bipolar disorder, schizophrenia, delusional disorders, dementia, anorexia nervosa, bulimia
Other	Medication side effects, alcohol or substance abuse, heavy metal exposure, body weight fluctuation

The good news is that a careful clinical evaluation can usually find a concrete reason for a person's complaint of fatigue. The reasons for fatigue will be identified in two-thirds of patients, but for the remaining one-third the underlying causes will not be identified.[7] When evaluating patients with a complaint of fatigue, the clinical approach needs to be very detailed and thorough. The clinical evaluation of fatigue encompasses the following five key elements[8]:

1. Taking a detailed history: This involves figuring out the pertinent aspects of fatigue, such as its duration (recent, prolonged, or chronic), onset (sudden or progressive), length of time needed to recover from fatigue (short or long), type of fatigue (physical or mental), and discovering the patient's typical level of physical activity (active or sedentary).

2. Physical examination: Should cover all regions and systems in the body, such as the cardiovascular, head and neck, musculoskeletal, respiratory, and neurological. A thorough physical exam might help to identify organic causes of fatigue (for example, heart disease) or it might help the clinician find some unusual causes of fatigue (for example, multiple sclerosis or another type of neuromuscular disease).

3. Medication review and toxic exposures: Many medications, both prescription and over-the-counter, can cause fatigue. Some of the classes of medications known to induce fatigue include long-acting antihistamines, corticosteroids, neuroleptics, antiarrhythmics, antidepressants, antihypertensives, and even herbal remedies. Consideration for chronic or acute toxic environmental exposures (for example, carbon monoxide, lead, mercury, and arsenic) should be part of this evaluation as well.

4. Psychiatric assessment: Psychiatric disorders such as depression, panic disorder, and even somatization (when bodily symptoms are due to psychological reasons) disorder need to be considered. Additionally, it is paramount that alcohol use/abuse and drug abuse are also discussed in the evaluation of fatigue.

5. Sleep disorder assessment: Sleep apnea (when breathing repeatedly stops for short periods during sleep), excessive sleepiness, and other problems with sleep need to be addressed when evaluating fatigue.

The workup of fatigue should also include an initial battery of laboratory tests to determine if an underlying cause can be identified.[9]

- Complete Blood Count—Anemia, infection
- Erythrocyte Sedimentation Rate or C-Reactive Protein—Inflammation
- Blood Urea Nitrogen—Kidney function
- Albumin—Liver's ability to synthesize compounds
- Electrolytes—Adequate amounts of sodium, potassium, etc.
- Creatinine (with estimation of glomerular filtration rate)—Kidney function
- Liver Transaminase Levels—Liver enzymes
- Thyroid-Stimulating Hormone Level—Over- or underactive thyroid function

- Fasting Plasma Glucose (Blood Sugar) Level—Diabetes
- Antinuclear Antibody Test—Autoimmune disease (e.g., lupus)
- Rheumatoid Factor Test—Autoimmune disease (rheumatoid arthritis)
- Urinalysis (dipstick only)—Diabetes, infection, kidney function
- Ferritin Level—Iron stores in the body
- Urine Pregnancy Test (women of childbearing age)—Pregnancy

When the clinical workup does not identify a cause, the diagnosis might end up being chronic fatigue syndrome. CFS is highly considered when fatigue has persisted for longer than 6 months.[10]

Diagnostic Criteria for CFS

The diagnosis of chronic fatigue syndrome is based on criteria established by the CDC.[11]

1. Chronic fatigue lasting longer than 6 months, not due to ongoing exertion, is not considerably relieved by rest, is of new onset and not lifelong, and results in substantial reduction in prior levels of activity.
2. Four or more of the following symptoms are present for six months or more:
   - Impaired memory or concentration
   - Postexertional malaise
   - Unrefreshing sleep
   - Muscle pain
   - Multi-joint pain without swelling or redness
   - Headaches
   - Sore throat that is frequent or recurring
   - Tender lymph nodes

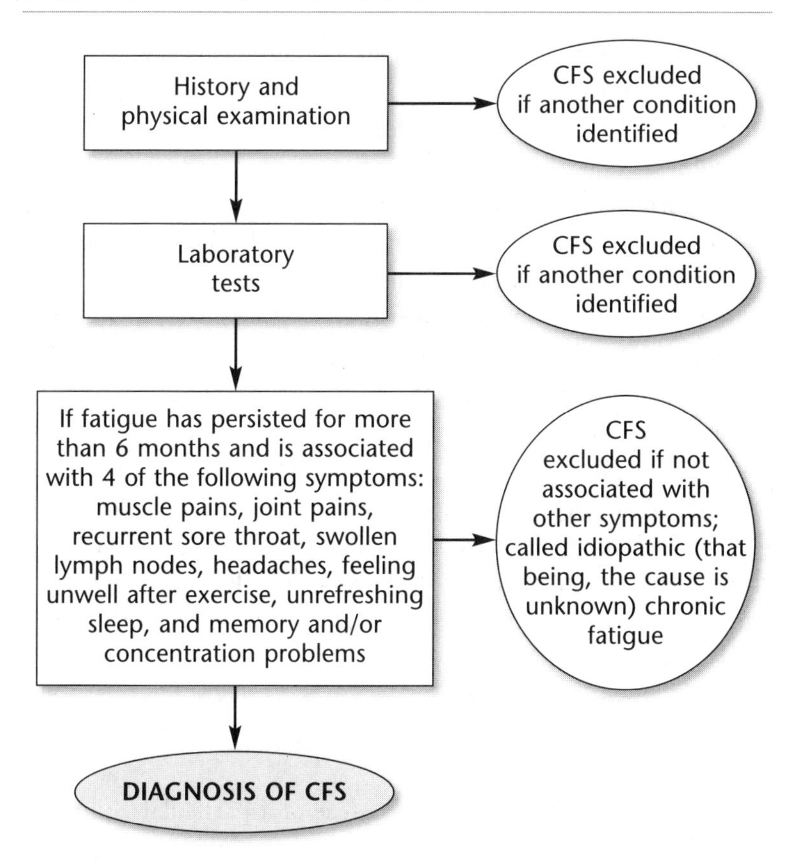

Case History

A seventy-year-old man presented at my clinical practice in October 2008 with concerns that he had chronic fatigue syndrome. He described a history of persistent symptoms that began during his childhood and included dizziness, and feeling dazed, heavy, sluggish, and tired. He also reported difficulties with memory and concentration, impaired mental dexterity, and being nervous all the time. As a child, he went to boarding school, which he found very painful due to the anxieties and humiliations he experienced when he had to speak in front of class. He also went through many life-changing events, including a technical education in a field that he had no passion for, several failed businesses, a difficult divorce, estrangement from his daughter, and legal problems with a former business partner. According to him, "There appears a paralysis of will; every course of action seems beset with insurmountable difficulties."

I performed a complete physical examination, and no neurological or muscular deficits were found. Physically, he was a healthy and vital man, so there was no need to pursue further diagnostic testing. After evaluating him over several office visits, I explained to him that he did not have CFS. An aspect of his history was inconsistent with a diagnosis of CFS—he reported benefiting both physically and psychologically from daily intense physical exercise. Every patient with CFS that I have evaluated has been worsened by physical activity and always requires several days or longer to recover. Instead of CFS, this patient's diagnosis was consistent with chronic depression or major depressive disorder. This case highlights the need for a thorough clinical evaluation when there is a chief complaint of fatigue.

Causes of Chronic Fatigue Syndrome

Doctors attempt to determine the cause of a particular condition in order to properly treat it. If a patient presents with fever, coughing, difficulty breathing, chest pain, an absence of breath sounds at the lung bases, and an overall sick appearance, the likely diagnosis would be pneumonia. This label, however, does not help with the identification of a cause. Once the ill patient undergoes further testing, such as a chest x-ray and blood tests, it is possible to determine the type of pneumonia. If testing demonstrates the presence of bacteria, the diagnosis would be changed to bacterial pneumonia and antibiotics would be prescribed.

Unfortunately, no diagnostic or laboratory tests have been found that identify the cause of chronic fatigue.[12] We have numerous theories about the possible causes of CFS, and yet not a single one has been fully endorsed by medical science as the principal cause of this elusive and life-altering syndrome. Research has shown that a combination of the following factors is implicated in the development of CFS: allergies, autonomic and central nervous system dysfunctions, environmental toxic exposures, an imbalanced immune system, infections, mental health problems, muscular dysfunctions, oxidative stress, and red blood cell abnormalities.

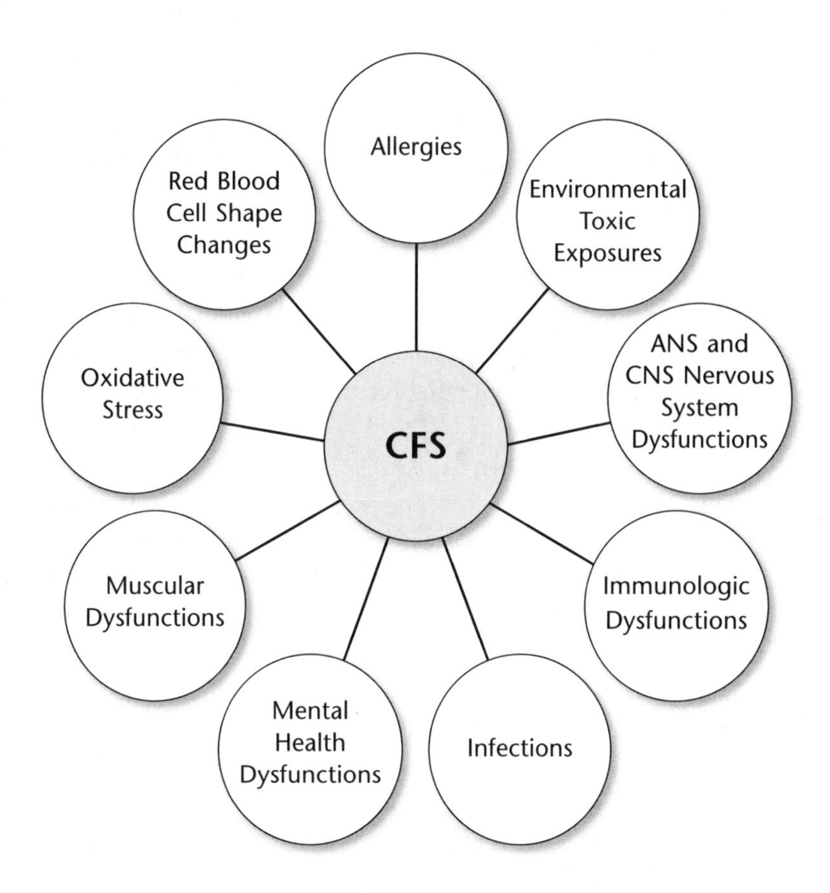

Allergies

Patients with chronic fatigue have a greater prevalence of allergies than the normal population.[13] CFS patients might be more vulnerable to atopic (allergic) illnesses such as allergic rhinitis (nose-related allergies) than the general population[14], but the research findings have not always been so clear-cut. Considering atopic illnesses are usually inherited, this would imply a genetic component. Research has shown that CFS patients have increased levels of eosinophil cationic proteins compared to patients without CFS.[15] Eosinophils are specialized white blood cells that are activated when triggered by allergies. Other research has not demonstrated that CFS patients are more subject to atopic illnesses than the general population when testing for specific antibodies (serum immunoglobulin E levels).[16]

If allergic rhinitis is, in fact, common among CFS patients, it could explain some of the persistent symptoms that characterize this syndrome, particularly chronic nasal congestion, which causes sleep disturbances and daytime fatigue. However, the relationship between allergic rhinitis and CFS is not so straightforward. Published data demonstrates that among the CFS population, 24 percent had no significant rhinitis complaints, 30 percent had positive skin tests suggesting the potential for allergic rhinitis, and 46 percent had nonallergic rhinitis.[17]

What about food intolerances? The majority of CFS patients complain about having reactions or sensitivities to foods. It is estimated that food intolerances are a significant factor in 20–30 percent of CFS cases and might be the primary trigger in 5–10 percent of cases.[18] One large study assessed the value of an elimination diet and did show improvements when CFS patients were placed on a diet free of provoking foods and chemicals.[19] The elimination diet consisted of a stringent diet without naturally occurring salicylates, biogenic amines, glutamate, and food additives for a period of 2–6 weeks. It might have also involved the avoidance of milk, wheat, and/or eggs. After the period of avoidance, patients were challenged with purified, graded doses of food substances at 48-hour intervals to ascertain reactions. Of the 966 patients who were evaluated for food and chemical reactions, about one-third satisfied the criteria for a diagnosis of CFS. From the 966 patients, 656 reported subjective improvements from following a strict elimination diet. In another study, 102 CFS patients responded to a questionnaire that evaluated their responses to an elimination diet: thirty-nine patients stated that the elimination diet made them feel "much better" or "completely well," twenty-five felt "a little better," and thirty-eight patients felt "no better at all."[20]

What all of these studies highlight are the complexities involved when evaluating CFS patients for allergies. Nevertheless, it is very likely that patients with CFS unduly suffer from allergic rhinitis and/or intolerances to foods and chemicals, which no doubt play a significant role in many of their chronic, debilitating symptoms.

Autonomic and Central Nervous System Dysfunctions

Patients with CFS exhibit nervous system impairments as evidenced by cognitive deficits in concentration, attention, and short-term memory.[21] Some of these cognitive deficits might result from abnormalities in the autonomic nervous system (ANS), which maintains balance (homeostasis) in the body by regulating various physiological activities that function unconsciously—the regulation of heart rate, digestive processes, respiration rate, salivation, perspiration, pupil size, urination, and sexual arousal.

In CFS, the ANS has problems properly regulating the flow of blood throughout the body, especially when standing is involved. When healthy people go from sitting to standing, or stand for prolonged periods of time, the ANS ensures that blood pressure is maintained so that there is adequate perfusion of blood into the brain. For CFS patients, on the other hand, it is common to become symptomatic (for example, feeling light-headed and fatigued) in response to standing.[22] Even though some studies have failed to find similar problems between the ANS and blood flow in CFS[23], it appears that for many patients the ANS cannot maintain proper blood flow in response to changes in posture. This would explain the presence of cognitive deficits among CFS patients, since cognitive processes depend on sufficient blood flow to the brain.

In addition to the ANS, the central nervous system (CNS) seems to be underfunctioning, leading to many of the cognitive disturbances associated with CFS. The CNS is the master controller of the entire nervous system and houses the brain and spinal cord. When CFS patients were examined with magnetic resonance imaging (MRI), lesions in the white matter of the brain were identified.[24] This is significant since the frontal lobes, which reside in the white matter of the brain, are involved in memory and in reactions to emotional events.

Another study using a specialized diagnostic imaging technique found impaired brain blood flow among CFS patients but not among normal subjects.[25] A study revealed altered frontal brain metabolism among patients with CFS or depression but not among normal subjects.[26] A more recent study found reduced absolute brain blood flow in rather broad areas among CFS patients compared to healthy individuals.[27] Based on these studies, it appears that CFS patients have derangements in both brain blood flow and metabolism, which helps to explain why they experience ongoing cognitive impairments such as memory and concentration disturbances. Despite these well-known facts, CFS patients face considerable frustration since these real and significant neurological dysfunctions are not obvious enough to be discovered on physical examination by a medical practitioner.[28]

Environmental Toxic Exposures

Toxic agents can produce an illness that would be clinically indistinguishable from chronic fatigue. For example, exposure to toxigenic molds leads to a myriad of symptoms that mimic CFS.[29] Other research has demonstrated an association between CFS and organochlorine and organophosphate exposures. Organochlorines are organic chemicals (containing chlorine and usually several other elements) that are used in herbicides, insecticides, fungicides, and polychlorinated biphenyls.[30] Organophosphates are also used for both domestic and industrial purposes, including in insecticides, nerve gases, ophthalmic (eye) agents, antiparasitic agents, and herbicides.[31] One study found that a group of CFS patients had higher total organochlorine levels compared to a group of normal individuals.[32] Another study found that CFS patients had significantly higher serum levels of the organochlorine compound 1,1-dichloro-2,2-bis(p-chlorophenyl) ethane (DDE) compared to control subjects.[33] Low-dose exposure to organophosphates not only caused symptoms that mimicked CFS but also produced neurological and hormonal abnormalities that were common among sufferers of CFS.[34]

When CFS patients with a toxic exposure history were compared to CFS patients without such a history, investigators discovered some interesting findings. Both groups of patients exhibited the same disturbances of hypothalamic function (the gland that helps to regulate the hormonal system), while the toxic-exposed group of CFS patients had more profound immunological abnormalities.[35]

Exposure to environmental toxins is potentially a triggering factor in some or many cases of chronic fatigue. Although it is impossible to know what percentage of CFS cases are directly caused by environmental toxins, the fact remains that some individuals are more vulnerable to toxins and end up developing this devastating medical syndrome. The precise biochemical factors that cause some CFS patients to be more vulnerable to environmental toxins continue to be the subject of much debate and investigation.

Imbalanced Immune System

Derangement in immune function has long been considered an underlying factor in the development of chronic fatigue. When patients are treated with specific immune-modulating medications (known as cytokines), such as interleukin-2 and alpha-interferon, they develop symptoms that mimic CFS.[36] When given in high doses to individuals without CFS, these two specific cytokines produce common CFS symptoms, such as disabling fatigue, muscle pain, and cognitive impairment. These types of reports give credibility to the idea that CFS might be an illness of immune system dysfunction.

Other reports implicate cells of the immune system known as natural killer (NK) cells in the immunological dysfunction associated with CFS. NK cells are vital in our ability to fend off viral infections. While the number of NK cells have not been shown to be deficient among CFS patients, these specialized cells do not function properly among those with chronic fatigue.[37] It has been hypothesized that a triggering event (for example, a viral infection) could, through a complex series of immunological and other physiological events, lead to chronic immune system abnormalities and ongoing symptoms of chronic fatigue.[38]

Infections

Many chronic fatigue sufferers link the onset of their illness to an acute flu-like infection. This is the subject of much controversy, since research has not fully supported the notion that an infectious agent (such as a virus) triggers the onset of CFS.[39] Yet, it is known that infectious agents causing mononucleosis, Lyme disease, Q fever, and a host of other diseases trigger CFS.[40] There is even research demonstrating that a subset of CFS patients (28 percent in one study) were infected with the parasite *Giardia lamblia*.[41] The current understanding is that the cause of CFS is not one infectious agent, but rather that the chronic immune system abnormalities that characterize CFS were probably initiated by a virus.[42]

Mental Health Problems

People with chronic fatigue are more prone to depression than are healthy individuals and they also tend to be highly sensitive people.[43] Furthermore, two-thirds of those with chronic fatigue have signs of major depressive illness, and half of all CFS patients have experienced at least one episode of major depression.[44] Given this information, it is easy to understand why some clinicians think that chronic fatigue is simply an offshoot of major depression. However, key features of CFS, such as sore throat, swollen lymph nodes, and feeling unwell after exercise, are normally absent among individuals with major depression. In addition, people with chronic fatigue do not routinely experience guilt, do not lack the ability to derive pleasure in everyday life, nor do they have a decrease in their motivation to do things, all of which are typical features of depressed patients.[45]

One study concluded that chronic fatigue is under-diagnosed in more than 80 percent of the people who have it and is very often misdiagnosed as depression.[46] Thus, there appears to be more differences than commonalities between CFS and major depression. This does not exclude the possibility, however, that some of the factors that predispose individuals to CFS might be mental in nature. Furthermore, many CFS patients also struggle with chronic anxiety, depression, and other mental health problems.

Muscular Dysfunctions

People with chronic fatigue typically complain of muscle aches and pains (myalgias). Compared to healthy individuals, patients with CFS have a reduced ability to perform muscular work.[47] A study found that those with CFS experience declines in cognitive function when performing maximal physical work compared to healthy individuals.[48] I have personally observed that many chronic fatigue patients also have a musculoskeletal condition known as fibromyalgia syndrome. The clinical features that characterize fibromyalgia syndrome are very similar to those of CFS, except that fibromyalgia is characterized by widespread pain in specific areas of the body, referred to as tender points. The specific diagnosis of fibromyalgia syndrome primarily involves the presence of widespread pain for at least 3 months duration in combination with at least eleven of eighteen specific tender points that occur on both sides of the body.[49]

Although many clinicians feel that chronic fatigue and fibromyalgia are separate illnesses, I believe them to be part of a similar clinical syndrome. Both conditions are marked by joint pains, weakness, fatigue, stiffness, numbness and tingling, poor sleep, and difficulty thinking clearly. Research supports the idea that both CFS and fibromyalgia syndrome might belong to the same clinical entity.[50]

Oxidative Stress

An emerging area of chronic fatigue research focuses on oxidative stress as an underlying factor. Oxidative stress refers to reactions in the body that result from breathing oxygen. When we breathe oxygen, we generate a group of "bad" chemicals called free radicals. In healthy individuals, there are adequate amounts of "good" chemicals called antioxidants to stop these free radicals from causing damage to our cells and other vital cellular components. However, individuals with CFS have a decline in their antioxidant systems so that they cannot adequately handle oxidative stress.[51] Individuals vulnerable to CFS and related conditions mount an increased and excessive production of nitric oxide and peroxynitrite when exposed to environmental toxins.[52] Peroxynitrite is a dangerous free radical that causes two detrimental side effects in the body: (1) it depletes cellular energy and leads to fatigue, and (2) it allows unwanted chemicals and other substances to enter the brain.[53]

The net result of these hazardous biochemical events include oxidative stress, overwhelmed antioxidant systems, nervous system dysfunction, increased sensitivity to environmental toxic exposures, and symptoms of chronic fatigue. Other researchers have also speculated that impaired antioxidant defenses and oxidative stress are prominent features of CFS.[54] Specific antioxidants like selenium, alpha-lipoic acid, and glutathione can be used therapeutically to stop the damage imposed by free radicals and help in the management of chronic fatigue.[55]

Red Blood Cell Abnormalities

Another theory that helps to explain the numerous clinical features of CFS involves red blood cell shape changes. Red blood cells (RBCs) are vital to our survival since they transport oxygen to all tissues and bodily organs. Normal RBCs are disc-shaped, which allows them to function properly within the body. Their diameters are greater than our smallest blood vessels (capillaries), so for RBCs to ensure adequate blood flow and oxygen to all of our tissues, they need to deform their shapes to traverse the capillaries. Their disc-shaped structure allows them to accomplish this remarkable feat. Researchers have demonstrated that the wide range of symptoms that characterizes chronic fatigue might result from impaired capillary blood flow.[56] A greater percentage of abnormally shaped RBCs occur among patients with CFS compared to healthy individuals or people suffering from multiple sclerosis.[57]

Thus, the symptoms of chronic fatigue could be directly related to the high percentage of abnormally shaped RBCs and their inability to deliver adequate amounts of oxygen to the tissues of the body.

Summary

Many things can contribute to the temporary experience of feeling fatigued. If fatigue lasts longer than it should, medical attention is required to determine if there are identifiable reasons for it. When specific causes cannot be found and when the fatigue persists longer than six months, a diagnosis of chronic fatigue syndrome is considered. If other symptoms such as muscle pain, multi-joint pain, sore throat, and unrefreshing sleep accompany the fatigue, a diagnosis of CFS is usually made.

Many factors have been considered as potential triggers or causes of CFS. While each of these individual factors has been the subject of numerous research reports, no single cause has been identified as the central culprit in triggering chronic fatigue. I believe that several of these factors will eventually be found to play a more dominant role in causing chronic fatigue. Perhaps at that time, more effective diagnostic tests will be developed to help clinicians sort through all the possible causes of CFS.

CHAPTER 2

LIFESTYLE MODIFICATIONS

According to general practitioner Dr. Erik T. Paterson, chronic fatigue syndrome (CFS) usually starts with a "stressed" organism. The stress, he explains, is hastened by several distinctive personality traits: having a type A personality, working much too hard, and never refusing to take on additional responsibilities—the kind of individual, as Dr. Paterson states, "that no civilization can do without."[1] The overarching problem is that these individuals become weakened and are thus more vulnerable to other insults, such as toxic environmental chemicals (obtained from food, air, and water) and even viruses.

Some of these individuals will unfortunately end up developing CFS and must learn how to bring proper balance into their lives; otherwise, progress will not be possible. How can patients with CFS bring more balance into their lives? Numerous experts in the field of chronic fatigue evaluated the evidence and summarized effective lifestyle and self-help strategies that can benefit those with CFS.[2] Here is a summary of the most important findings.

Learn to Recognize Early Warning Signs and Prevent Crashes

Mindfulness exercises help people with chronic fatigue to understand the impact of their activities and environment on their mind, body, and emotional states, particularly given the persistent nature of CFS. This allows you to understand the early warning signs and the need to quickly intervene when experiencing excessive fatigue and/or sensory stimulation, information overload, pressure from life that is too fast-paced, excessive stress, the inability to organize tasks, and so on.

Use Stress Reduction and Relaxation Techniques

Breathing and meditative practices are encouraged, as these techniques move awareness into the present. They should be done in a quiet place and should be basic enough that they do not increase fatigue or stress. These techniques can be used not only to reduce the burden that physical and mental stress has upon those suffering from CFS, but also as an effective strategy in periods of excessive sensory and motor stimulation.

Employ Energy Conservation Techniques to Reduce the Strains of Daily Activities

Energy conservation techniques include the use of kitchen gadgets to help when opening jars, easier food preparation techniques, less physical ways of getting laundry done, and so on. In other words, use all available resources to reduce the strains of maintaining a household.

Modify Your Environment

Modifying the environment simply means restructuring and reorganizing the placement of furniture, appliances, and other household items in order to minimize the emotional and physical burden that results from doing household chores. This same idea should be adopted into your workplace to simplify the tasks that might otherwise worsen chronic fatigue symptoms.

Limit and/or Avoid Known Triggers

Potential triggers for chronic fatigue include:

- Viral infections
- Changes in sleep schedule
- Cold exposure
- Overexertion (physical or mental)
- Prolonged muscular or mental activity
- Sensory overload of any type (visual, auditory, etc.)
- Information overload
- Excessive stress
- Prolonged driving
- Air travel (due to jet lag, re-circulated stale air and viruses, stimulation of the inner ear apparatus, and excessive vibration)

Practice Self-Development

Personal development can be encouraged by:

- Setting aside time for oneself
- Trusting inner feelings and experiences
- Setting emotional and personal boundaries
- Extending emotional boundaries when possible so that situations that used to give rise to anxiety or "crashes" become more tolerable and less disabling
- Extending perceptual and cognitive boundaries by engaging in games, puzzles, and other activities that help to improve memory and gently extend one's limits of cognitive tolerability

Optimize Sleep Hygiene

- Pace your daytime activities
- Establish a regular bedtime
- Use the bed for sleeping only and not for other activities like watching television
- Ensure that the sleep environment is dark and quiet
- Make the bedroom a "worry free" zone
- Use a supportive mattress and pillow and other measures such as a contoured pillow or a pillow between the legs
- Use sleep aids (natural supplements or drugs), when necessary

Use Appropriate Body Movement and Fitness Techniques

- Adopt good body mechanics when sitting, standing, driving, and so on
- Improve your balance
- Use daily activities to stay active
- Don't overdo your household chores and other daily duties
- Maintain an effective but not destabilizing exercise routine

Establishing a regular exercise routine is an important strategy in overcoming CFS. There is a tendency for CFS patients to overdo exercise and "crash." Exercise must be restricted to non-fatigue types of activity and should not exceed your energy levels.[3] Otherwise, you'll feel worse and your progress significantly slows down. Prior to engaging in an exercise program, you should undergo a thorough physical evaluation, including assessing for the appropriateness of the exercise program, cardiovascular function and risk factors, joint function and the presence of osteoarthritis, muscle function, medication use, concomitant problems that might reduce the effectiveness or usefulness of exercise, and your current level of physical fitness.[4]

An effective exercise program must include all of the following elements if it is to be useful:

1. It must minimize muscle microtrauma: Use exercises that have minimal movement requirements and that emphasize elongation (e.g., overhead movements).

2. It must minimize central sensitization: Use appropriate types of exercises that do not cause pain and injury. The intensity of the various exercises needs to be kept to a minimum or else you will have a significant flare-up. The intensity needs to be furthered modified since those with CFS do not achieve the same maximum heart rates as do normal individuals.

3. It must maximize self-efficacy: In order to be more autonomous, stick with an exercise program that does not extend beyond your limits. The frequency and duration of exercise can be gradually increased over the course of many months, but the level of intensity must always remain low.

4. The individual exercise program must include:
   - An adequate warm-up and cool-down period to prevent injuries.
   - Strength-training exercises to increase the size of the muscles and to improve joint stability, with the focus being on the upper and lower body, the abdominal area, and the muscles along the spine.
   - Endurance exercises involving non-impact activities, such as walking or gentle exercises done in a heated pool.
   - Stretching maneuvers to improve flexibility and to reduce the pain associated with tight muscles.
   - Appropriate pacing and balance—be sure to stay well hydrated with water and electrolytes taken prior to exercise and your exercise program should be undertaken in a very gradual fashion.

Summary

In order to recover from chronic fatigue, you must adopt new ways of living. This involves: (1) understanding early warning signs so that crashes are prevented; (2) using stress reduction and relaxation techniques to reduce tension and bring awareness into the present; (3) conserving energy by relying on kitchen gadgets and other resources to reduce the strains of maintaining a household; (4) making environmental modifications to minimize the emotional and physical burden of completing the tasks of daily living; (5) limiting and/or avoiding known environmental triggers such as viral infections, overexertion, and air travel; (6) working on self-development by setting aside time for yourself and instituting appropriate emotional and personal boundaries; (7) optimizing sleep hygiene; and (8) using appropriate body movement and fitness techniques to improve physical capacity. A regular exercise program should ideally lead to more self-reliance and autonomy, and the intensity level should always remain low.

In my clinical experience with chronic fatigue patients, these lifestyle modifications allow for a more enjoyable quality of life with fewer symptoms. They can help you achieve more balance and pacing in your daily routine. However, if these lifestyle modifications are not maintained, the chances of recovery are very slim.

CHAPTER 3

TREATING ALLERGIES

Dietary modifications can play a major role in improving quality of life for those with chronic fatigue syndrome (CFS). There is emerging evidence suggesting a link between adverse reactions to foods or diet-derived compounds (food allergies) and the development of CFS.[1] An elimination diet can help provide relief, as can vitamin C and other nutrients.

Food Allergies and Chronic Fatigue

One investigator reported less fatigue in 73 percent of CFS patients who implemented dietary modifications.[2] This finding is important since fatigue is the central problem in CFS. Other research demonstrated a reduction in the inflammatory compounds called cytokines when food intolerances were eliminated by dietary modifications.[3] When individuals with food intolerances were challenged with dairy and wheat, cytokine levels were significantly elevated. This can cause a myriad of symptoms that mimic the features of chronic fatigue, such as headaches, muscle pains, joint pains, and gastrointestinal disturbances.

When CFS patients eliminated wheat, milk, benzoates, nitrites, nitrates, and food colorings and other additives from their diets, 90 percent experienced symptom reduction in fatigue, recurrent fever, sore throat, muscle pain, headache, joint pain, and cognitive dysfunction.[4] There was also a reduction in irritable bowel symptoms, which is particularly relevant since the prevalence of irritable bowel syndrome is high among those with CFS.[5] In another study in which CFS patients eliminated food intolerances, there was complete alleviation of chronic fatigue in twenty patients.[6]

The worst or most implicated foods were milk, wheat, and corn. This is interesting because wheat, dairy, corn, and eggs are the most common allergens and are known to trigger numerous symptoms and exacerbations of diseases such as arthritis, eczema, inflammatory bowel disease, irritable bowel syndrome, and migraines.[7] In one study, 70 percent of sixty-four CFS patients experienced improvements in their physical symptoms and mental outlook when they followed a wheat-free diet in addition to nutrient supplementation and homeopathy.[8] Alcohol is another dietary trigger common to CFS patients. One study determined that 60 percent of CFS patients noted alcohol intolerance as the onset of their chronic fatigue.[9]

How Dietary Intolerances Lead to Chronic Fatigue

It is clear that people with chronic fatigue are subject to numerous food allergies. There are three related mechanisms by which dietary intolerances cause disturbances in function:

- Direct pharmacological effects of substances found in foods or beverages
- Hidden allergic responses to foods or beverages
- Intestinal hyperpermeability (leaky gut syndrome)

Direct Pharmacological Effects of Substances Found in Foods or Beverages

The main culprits in this category are caffeine, alcohol, and sugar (sucrose). Caffeine is a stimulant and a widely used psychoactive substance that can sometimes trigger many symptoms. Common bodily manifestations of caffeinism (in descending order of frequency) are sweating, insomnia, withdrawal headache, diarrhea, anxiety, increased heart rate, and tremulousness.[10] Caffeine has also been shown to cause both anxiety and depressive symptoms.[11] Side effects from caffeine consumption are not uncommon. In a published case report, caffeine use was associated with symptoms such as light-headedness, tremulousness, breathlessness, headache, and disturbances in heart function (premature ventricular contractions).[12] These symptoms ceased once the caffeine was discontinued and recurred on two separate occasions when caffeine was re-challenged after periods of abstinence. Vulnerable CFS patients are prone to experience exacerbations when consuming any amount of caffeine. I have observed that the severity of chronic fatigue seems to correlate with the amount of caffeine consumed. Even one cup of coffee can be problematic for people who are susceptible. To make matters worse, people who habitually consume caffeine are prone to withdrawal symptoms that can mimic many features of CFS. It is paramount that people with chronic fatigue avoid caffeine at all times.

People with CFS tend to be intolerant of alcohol and its consumption provokes symptoms. Alcohol inhibits the production of blood sugar (the brain's main fuel source) and increases the production of lactic acid (which causes muscle pain).[13] Alcohol has also been shown to increase anxiety[14], which frequently accompanies CFS. Like caffeine withdrawal, discontinuing alcohol can cause anxiety and hyperventilation[15], which will only worsen symptoms of CFS. If you have chronic fatigue, it is best to avoid consuming alcohol.

Refined sugar should also be avoided, as its consumption can trigger emotional reactions and provoke symptoms in susceptible individuals. Refined sugar is white or table sugar, which comes from sugar cane, sugar beets, and sugar maples, and is the most commonly consumed sugar. It is found in many commonly consumed, processed food items, such as ketchup, candy bars, pastries, canned fruits and vegetables, ice cream, frozen pizza, and peanut butter. In the body, refined sugars are broken down to glucose, which is the brain's main fuel source. When people with CFS eat refined sugar, it results in surges of blood glucose, which subsequently leads to sharp drops in blood sugar, referred to as hypoglycemic episodes.

Even though the body has many overlapping mechanisms to guard against hypoglycemia, the habitual ingestion of refined sugar puts stress on these systems. The end result is poor blood sugar regulation, which often leads to more unhealthy eating behaviors, more stress, and numerous flare-ups or "crashes."

Studies have demonstrated that glucose infusions induce panic attacks and increase blood lactate concentrations in patients with anxiety.[16] I have observed similar reactions among CFS patients who continue to eat refined sugars despite my constant encouragement to stop. Anxiety is a common problem that those with CFS struggle with.[17] When people with CFS chronically consume sugar, they experience increased anxiety and sometimes panic attacks, which may be accompanied by more muscle pain. The blood glucose surges lead to increased blood lactate, which is biochemically responsible for the sensation of muscle pain.

Hidden Allergic Responses to Foods or Beverages

Hidden allergies can be loosely defined as reactions to foods occurring many hours after, or several days following, the ingestion of the allergenic foods.[18] Foods that are most commonly associated with hidden allergic reactions include the following:

- Dairy products
- Wheat, barley, and rye
- Eggs
- Corn
- Chocolate
- Tea and coffee
- Sugar
- Yeast
- Soy
- Citrus fruits
- Beef and pork
- Tomato
- Peanuts and nuts
- Seafood

Many people with chronic fatigue are unaware that their continued ill-health is related to what they have been habitually consuming. Symptoms reported by several patients after consuming common food allergens include[19]:

Wheat: Restless, yawning and unable to concentrate, frontal headache, visual blurring, nausea, abdominal pain, muscle spasm, and back pain described as "colon spasm."

Milk: Irritable, restless, sharp abdominal cramps, bloating with visible distention, nervous, tired, dizziness, confusion, and sore throat.

Egg: Intermittent fatigue, nervous, unable to concentrate, coughing, generalized itching, and nausea.

Corn: Frontal headache, visual blurring, fatigue, sore throat, abdominal pain, difficulty concentrating, and feeling irritable and miserable.

Leaky Gut Syndrome

The gut (small intestine) normally protects itself by not allowing the absorption of allergy-provoking (antigenic) or disease-causing (pathogenic) molecules and by maintaining a healthy immune response.[20] When these properties are compromised, as in leaky gut syndrome, unwanted proteins and other molecules from the intestinal tract enter the bloodstream and cause numerous symptoms. One of the common causes of leaky gut is food intolerances[21], since adverse reactions to foods have been shown to cause gut leakiness.[22] Recall that one of the consequences of a food allergy is an increase in inflammatory compounds known as cytokines. Cytokines compromise the intestinal tract, creating "leakiness" between the cells of the small intestine.[23] The symptoms of leaky gut syndrome mimic many symptoms of CFS and can include abdominal pain, chronic joint and muscle pain, confusion, fuzzy thinking, gas, indigestion, mood swings, nervousness, poor immunity, recurrent infections, skin rashes, diarrhea, bedwetting, poor memory, shortness of breath, constipation, bloating, aggressive behavior, anxiety, fatigue, and feeling toxic.[24]

Dietary Solutions

Because pharmacological reactions to foods, hidden allergies, and leaky gut syndrome are so prevalent, I have all my CFS patients complete a seven-day diet diary to see how regularly they are consuming common food allergens, how frequently they are eating suspected foods in a given day, and the quantities consumed. They report any symptoms that are increased or alleviated by ingesting certain foods. Once the seven-day diet diary has been received, I analyze it and assess if the symptoms are related to foods chronically consumed. If the diet diary implicates some of the common food allergens (as it usually does), I recommend an oligoantigenic (elimination) diet, followed by individual food challenges to pinpoint which specific foods are involved in producing symptoms.[25]

An oligoantigenic diet contains as few allergens as possible.[26] You need to stay on the diet for at least 3–4 weeks. Symptoms of food withdrawal tend to occur during the first few days of the diet while patients pass through an addiction period. Significant improvements typically occur after 3–4 weeks. If symptoms persist, it is likely that some of the foods on the elimination diet are themselves provoking reactions. When this happens, an alternative oligoantigenic diet should be tried for an additional 2–3 weeks to see if many of the symptoms clear.

SAMPLE OLIGOANTIGENIC DAILY DIET

Breakfast	Lunch	Dinner
Lamb	Turkey	Chicken
Potatoes	Rice	Potatoes
Pear	Banana	Apple
Broccoli	Cauliflower	Collard greens
Sunflower oil	Sunflower oil	Sunflower oil
Water or mineral water	Water or mineral water	Water or mineral water
Calcium gluconate (1 gram)	Calcium gluconate (1 gram)	Calcium gluconate (1 gram)
Vitamins (as prescribed)	Vitamins (as prescribed)	Vitamins (as prescribed)

Once you have experienced significant symptomatic relief, it is time to do food challenges by testing individual foods one at a time and every four days. For example, to test milk, you would consume 1–2 glasses at breakfast, 1–2 glasses at lunch, and 1–2 glasses at dinner. Record any symptoms that occur immediately after ingesting the challenged food and also record any symptoms that arise over the next three days as well. After the first day of the food challenge, no additional foods are to be challenged or tested until the three days have passed, due to the potential of delayed allergic reactions. If you have a severe allergic reaction to a tested food item, taking 1 teaspoon of buffered vitamin C three times daily will usually stop the reaction.

These allergic reactions are not to be confused with the potentially lethal allergic reaction known as anaphylaxis, which causes throat constriction due to swelling, hives, and loss of consciousness. These food reactions, on the other hand, are merely nuisance reactions that exacerbate symptoms of chronic fatigue, such as muscle pain, joint pain, and gastrointestinal disturbances. The oligoantigenic diet must be maintained throughout the testing or challenge period. This process is continued with other allergenic foods, one at a time, and typically takes 14–21 days to complete.

Once the challenge phase is completed, new daily food practices must be adopted. One way to effectively manage allergic reactions is to eliminate all implicated foods from your diet and never (knowingly) consume them again. Another method involves a rotation diet, during which the implicated foods can be consumed once every four days in order to limit possible allergic reactions.

Vitamin Solutions

The vitamin solutions for controlling food intolerances are sparse since dietary modifications are the mainstays of effective treatment.

Vitamin C

Vitamin C has an intimate relationship with histamine levels in the blood.[27] Histamine is released by specialized mast cells and causes many of the uncomfortable symptoms that characterize food intolerances. When vitamin C levels are low in the blood, histamine levels rise—therefore, consuming modest doses of vitamin C lowers blood histamine levels as a result of its antihistamine effects.

This cannot be achieved by consuming dietary sources of vitamin C, such as oranges, guavas, peppers, lemon juice, strawberries, and collard greens. Rather, you need to supplement with vitamin C. Therapeutic doses of 1,000–3,000 mg per day are helpful in lowering histamine, but to obtain good control over food allergies it is usually necessary to take daily amounts of vitamin C that are just below bowel tolerance (the amount of the vitamin that produces gas or diarrhea). To determine your bowel tolerance amount, take 1,000–4,000 mg of vitamin C every hour until you experience lots of gas or have diarrhea (neither of which are dangerous). If, for example, these nuisance effects occur after taking 12,000 mg of vitamin C, then your bowel tolerance has been achieved. Adjust your dose of vitamin C dose to an amount that is 500–1,000 mg below bowel tolerance.

The body needs large quantities of vitamin C when under stress, meaning that the bowel tolerance doses can be much more than the 12,000 mg cited here. Side effects are rare, but some patients with CFS have difficulty tolerating regular vitamin C (ascorbic acid) tablets or crystals. In these situations, other forms of vitamin C like sodium ascorbate, mineral ascorbates, or Ester C can be substituted.

Other Solutions

Glutamine

Glutamine is an amino acid derived from dietary protein. Supplemental glutamine is therapeutically useful since it heals the gut. Specifically, it increases the height and thickness of the small intestinal cells, improves immune function, and reduces the "leakiness" between the cells.[28] Numerous studies have demonstrated that glutamine possesses important healing properties that reduce the negative consequences of leaky gut syndrome.[29]

Therapeutic doses of glutamine are in the range of 10–40 grams per day, taken on an empty stomach with juice, either sixty minutes before or ninety minutes after a meal.[30] Glutamine has no adverse side effects associated with its use.

Probiotics

Billions of "friendly" bacteria, such as *Lactobacillus* and *Bifidobacteria,* live in both the small and large intestines to help with digestion, produce vitamins, and provide immune protection. Probiotics are a supplemental form of these bacteria that have been shown to reduce gut leakiness by strengthening the integrity of the cells of the small intestine and by reducing reactions triggered by allergenic foods.[31] A report suggested that the use of probiotics among people with chronic fatigue would reduce allergies, improve antioxidant status, and enhance the absorption of micronutrients.[32]

The use of probiotics can reduce symptoms of irritable bowel syndrome, a condition characterized by altered stool frequency (diarrhea alternating with constipation), altered stool form (hard or loose), altered stool passage (straining or urgency), and the passing of mucus. Probiotics improve the health of the large intestine and likely reduce toxic byproducts of poor digestion that contribute to symptoms as well.

Many clinical trials have been done on a variety of probiotic strains for the treatment of irritable bowel, so it is imperative that you work with your clinician to determine the most appropriate strains to use.[33] The starting dosage should be low, such as 100 million to 6 billion colony-forming units each day, and then can be increased gradually until you reach the most therapeutic dose. Patients with CFS might experience a brief worsening of their symptoms during the first few days of probiotic treatment.

Quercetin

Quercetin is a naturally occurring bioflavonoid found in apples and onions. It specifically stabilizes mast cells, reduces the release of histamine, and prevents food allergies from causing leakiness within the cells of the small intestine.[34] It is a local treatment, in that most of it remains within the small intestine and the rest of the gastrointestinal tract until it is eliminated through the bowels.[35]

Doses in the range of 400–500 mg of quercetin should be taken three times daily, about 15–20 minutes before meals. Higher dosages, in the range of 1,000–5,000 mg three times daily, might lead to better clinical outcomes.[36] Quercetin has not been associated with any adverse side effects.

Case History

A thirty-six-year-old woman presented to the Robert Schad Naturopathic Clinic, in Toronto, Canada, in September 2008. Her chief complaints were chronic depression and borderline personality disorder. She had an extensive history of mental health issues spanning several decades. After carefully evaluating her and monitoring her for about twelve months, it was determined that chronic fatigue syndrome provided a better explanation of her symptoms than did chronic depression or borderline personality disorder. We based this on her lengthy history of non-refreshing sleep, post-exercise malaise, fatigue spanning twelve months (and perhaps several decades), intermittent sore throats, chronic headaches and joint pains, and persistent cognitive disturbances affecting her concentration and memory.

Numerous treatments were tried, including chromium, vitamin B-complex, intramuscular injections of vitamin B_{12}, niacinamide, and melatonin, but without providing much relief. We then instituted an oligoantigenic diet that eliminated common allergens such as wheat and dairy. When she was on this diet, the majority of her symptoms improved, for she had noticeable positive changes in her mood, energy level, sleep, headaches, and concentration. During the challenge phase, the majority of her symptoms returned when she ingested wheat. It was rather obvious that wheat was the main trigger of her symptoms. She was instructed to follow a wheat-free diet and to examine food labels very carefully for hidden sources of wheat. She has made good progress since instituting these dietary changes and the vast majority of her chronic fatigue symptoms have improved.

Does this patient have chronic fatigue syndrome or does she have something that mimics it? At present, the patient's diagnosis is CFS, but she might actually have celiac disease, a condition characterized by the body's inability to tolerate the gluten component of wheat. Gluten is also found in other grains such as oats (often contaminated with gluten), barley, rye, malt, and buckwheat. Celiac disease is characterized by many symptoms that resemble CFS. The initial symptoms of celiac disease include memory disturbances and an awkward gait[37], common features of both celiac disease and CFS.[38] Also, there might be more celiac disease among CFS patients compared to the general population.[39] Plus, this patient had laboratory evidence showing very low iron stores, one of the first clues to arriving at a diagnosis of celiac disease.[40] Even though we have not run specific laboratory tests to confirm or eliminate celiac disease as a potential diagnosis, this case highlights the importance of having chronic fatigue patients undergo more specific testing for celiac disease when they have adverse reactions to wheat.

TREATMENTS FOR ALLERGIES

OLIGOANTIGENIC (ELIMINATION) DIET

THERAPEUTIC EFFECT: To identify and reduce dietary intolerances (food allergies)

DAILY DOSAGE: Follow a diet that does not contain any implicated dietary items, or a rotation diet in which the allergenic foods are ingested infrequently

VITAMIN C

THERAPEUTIC EFFECT: A natural antihistamine that reduces diet-related food reactions

DAILY DOSAGE: 1,000–3,000 mg; to optimally control diet-related food reactions, it may be necessary to increase the amount to just below bowel tolerance

GLUTAMINE

THERAPEUTIC EFFECT: An amino acid that nourishes the small intestine and reduces gut leakiness

DAILY DOSAGE: 10–40 grams

PROBIOTICS

THERAPEUTIC EFFECT: Replenishes the small and large intestines with beneficial bacteria that reduce both gut leakiness and symptoms of irritable bowel syndrome

DAILY DOSAGE: 100 million to 6 billion colony-forming units (can be gradually increased over time)

QUERCETIN

THERAPEUTIC EFFECT: Reduces the release of histamine from mast cells and prevents gut leakiness

DAILY DOSAGE: 400–5,000 mg with meals

Summary

With chronic fatigue, strict dietary modifications must be adopted, including avoidance of all caffeine, alcohol, and refined sugars. The habitual consumption of these items leads to metabolic consequences characterized by increased lactic acid levels in the blood and muscles and impaired circulation, all of which exacerbate the symptoms of CFS. Many people with CFS also suffer from food intolerances, which are often the result of hidden allergic reactions and leaky gut syndrome. To identify and effectively treat these allergies, those with chronic fatigue should complete an oligoantigenic (elimination) diet followed by individual food challenges. Once all implicated foods have been identified, they should be strictly avoided or only ingested once every four days to limit ongoing allergic reactions.

Although dietary modifications are the best way to improve reactions related to food intolerances, everyone with CFS should supplement with vitamin C due to its antihistamine properties. A select number of other treatments should also be considered:

- Glutamine—to improve the health of the gut
- Quercetin—to prevent reactions due to food intolerances
- Probiotics—to reduce symptoms of irritable bowel syndrome and prevent the accumulation of toxic byproducts of poor digestion.

CHAPTER 4

Optimizing Autonomic and Central Nervous System Function

People with chronic fatigue syndrome (CFS) suffer from nervous system impairments as a result of abnormalities in both their autonomic and central nervous systems. The autonomic nervous system (ANS) abnormalities lead to blood flow problems and even drops in blood pressure when standing, which can be responsible for symptoms such as light-headedness and fatigue. The central nervous system (CNS) abnormalities may involve alterations in brain blood flow and brain metabolism, which are presumed to be responsible for cognitive deficits involving concentration, attention, and short-term memory. I would also add mental fatigue and fogginess to the list of cognitive deficits that those with CFS experience. To remedy these nervous system disturbances, a number of nutritional options are available that can optimize the functioning of both the ANS and CNS.

Dietary Solutions

In the previous chapter, I recommended that people with chronic fatigue consider following an oligoantigenic (elimination) diet followed by a challenge phase to pinpoint dietary intolerances (food allergies). Once all implicated dietary items have been identified, they should be strictly avoided or ingested only once every four days to limit ongoing allergic reactions. This is a vital step when trying to recover from CFS.

Vitamin Solutions

Vitamins B_1, B_2, and B_6

Vitamins B_1 (thiamine), B_2 (riboflavin), and B_6 (pyridoxine) provide essential support to the nervous system and improve cognitive function. Among healthy individuals, deficits of these vitamins can lead to impairments in nervous system functioning. A study evaluated the relationship between vitamin status, psychological performance, and mental state in over 1,000 healthy men.[1] The thiamine-deficient individuals displayed poor memory and reaction performance indicative of cognitive deficits. A few unfavorable results were also found among men who were deficient in either pyridoxine or riboflavin. The overall results clearly showed an important association between unfavorable psychometric (psychological) findings and an insufficient supply of B vitamins. It also demonstrated that vitamin supplementation can lead to cognitive improvements in cases where there are documented B-vitamin deficiencies.

These three B vitamins were also evaluated in a study that involved patients with chronic fatigue.[2] Twelve patients with established CFS had their blood analyzed for deficiencies of thiamine, riboflavin, and pyridoxine. The results revealed functional deficiencies in these B vitamins, which were presumed to be related to low dietary intakes or to a gastrointestinal problem such as malabsorption. There was further speculation that these B-vitamin deficiencies might be responsible for specific CNS impairments that many patients with chronic fatigue suffer from, such as memory problems. While there are other B vitamins that support the nervous system (for example, folic acid and vitamins B_5 and B_{12}), it seems likely that these particular B vitamins might improve CNS function, especially when there are cognitive problems.

I encourage ingesting healthy dietary sources of these B vitamins, such as chicken, lamb, lentils, almonds, mushrooms, broccoli, and pine nuts. I also prescribe a B-complex 50 or 100, which means that the amounts of B vitamins in the supplement generally yield 50 or 100 mg of each. My patients take one B-complex 50 or 100 each day with a meal, and they might need to double the amount if no improvement in cognitive symptoms results after 4–8 weeks of use. B-complex vitamin supplements must be taken with meals or else nausea and rare cases of vomiting can occur. The urine will also appear much more yellow, but this has no negative consequence and is without any side effects. The yellow color simply means that the B vitamins have been absorbed (it reflects the amount of B_2 that has been filtered through the kidneys).

Supplemental riboflavin also helps in the prevention of migraine headaches, which unfortunately affect many people with CFS.[3] Migraine headaches are characterized by many symptoms, such as light-headedness, nausea, vomiting, sensitivities to noise and light, blind spots, flashing lights, and a throbbing headache. Clinical trials have proven that riboflavin is an effective vitamin treatment for migraine prevention.[4] In a randomized, controlled trial, the migraine patients taking riboflavin had a statistically significant reduction in their migraine attacks from four to two per month after three months of treatment.[5] If migraine headaches are a concern, I have my CFS patients take an additional 400 mg per day of riboflavin in addition to what they are getting from their B-complex supplement. There are no risks or side effects from taking additional riboflavin.

Vitamin B_3

In this section, I mention two specific forms of vitamin B_3, niacin (nicotinic acid) and nicotinamide adenine dinucleotide (NADH). Do not substitute these forms of B_3 for other readily available forms, such as non-flush niacin (inositol hexaniacinate) or niacinamide (nicotinamide). Niacin and NADH are the preferred forms when trying to alleviate the nervous system impairments that accompany chronic fatigue.

It is my contention that many people with CFS suffer from a vitamin B_3 dependency disorder. The term *dependency* simply means that those with chronic fatigue require much more vitamin B_3 than their daily diets provide (a typical daily diet generally contains 13–20 mg). This is not the same as having a "deficiency" in vitamin B_3 due to an inadequate diet, which would be caused by obtaining less than 20 mg each day of the vitamin. When the diet is deficient in vitamin B_3, the nutritional disease pellagra eventually develops, characterized by diarrhea, dermatitis, dementia, and eventually death. Pellagra reached epidemic proportions in the American South in the early 1900s, but it is uncommon today, except for rare cases among severely malnourished persons living on the street or among persons with severe wasting diseases. The reason for a vitamin B_3 dependency among those with CFS is unclear, but it would be caused by poor nutrition as well as environmental, genetic, and metabolic stresses.[6] The features that characterize a vitamin B_3 dependency resemble those of CFS, particularly the nervous system impairments.

COMPARISON OF VITAMIN B_3 DEPENDENCY AND CHRONIC FATIGUE

CLINICAL FEATURES OF VITAMIN B_3 DEPENDENCY	CLINICAL FEATURES OF CHRONIC FATIGUE SYNDROME
Cognitive disturbances and, in severe cases, dementia	Memory and concentration problems
Disordered thinking and thoughts	Brain fatigue and brain fog
Generalized fatigue	Chronic fatigue
Mood issues, such as depression and anxiety	Depression, anxiety, and other psychiatric issues
Muscle and joint aches and pains	Muscle and joint aches and pains
Diarrhea and constipation	Irritable bowel syndrome
Malabsorption	Possible malabsorption

Vitamin B_3 is an excellent "normalizer" of the nervous system and would help correct the ANS and CNS impairments that characterize chronic fatigue. Optimal therapeutic doses support the ANS and might reduce the blood flow problems and blood pressure drops that can result from standing. Vitamin B_3 also supports the CNS and might resolve cognitive impairments, such as memory problems and the associated brain fog/fatigue issues.

The NADH form of vitamin B_3 has been used therapeutically to treat chronic fatigue. NADH is the coenzyme of vitamin B_3, meaning it is the active form within the body. In a randomized, clinical pilot study, the use of supplemental NADH helped eight of twenty-six (31 percent) of CFS patients compared to only 8 percent in the placebo group.[7] In a follow-up study, 73 percent of the CFS patients from the previous study achieved marked improvement over time.[8] In another clinical study, the use of supplemental NADH produced statistically significant reductions in symptoms during the first three months of treatment compared to a group given psychotherapy and other nutritional supplements.[9]

There is evidence that the niacin form improves blood flow to the extremities of the body. Niacin causes peripheral vasodilation and skin flushing by inducing the production of a chemical in the skin known as prostaglandin D_2.[10] This effect might resolve the blood flow problems that underlie the ANS issues that many people with CFS experience. It is unknown if prostaglandin D_2 causes vasodilation within the brain, yet there is some evidence to suggest that it does lead to increased brain blood flow.[11] Reports from the 1950s demonstrated that niacin caused vasodilation of the cerebral (brain) blood vessels and that intravenous administration increased the rate of brain blood flow.[12] Unfortunately, there have not been more recent reports examining these effects. I believe that supplemental niacin would improve brain blood flow, which could prove therapeutic for the CNS impairments found in many with chronic fatigue.

An effective therapeutic dose of NADH is 10 mg daily, which might have to be increased to 20 mg if no improvements are observed after three months of use. While it might appear that the dose of NADH is similar to the amount of vitamin B_3 that is obtained from a typical diet (chicken, lamb, lentils, almonds, and mushrooms), because NADH is the active form, it is highly unlikely that people with CFS are producing adequate amounts of this coenzyme from dietary sources. Remember, CFS sufferers have a vitamin B_3 dependency disorder and will be unable to obtain optimal amounts of the vitamin from diet alone.

If the niacin form of vitamin B_3 is also desired, it must be used with a full understanding of its pharmacological properties. Niacin possesses important therapeutic properties that nourish the nervous system by correcting for a vitamin B_3 dependency and by increasing blood flow to the extremities and likely the brain. It achieves this by producing a flush that is not dangerous but can be uncomfortable to some individuals with CFS. The flush typically begins about 15–30 minutes after ingesting the vitamin and starts on the forehead, extending to the face, upper back, and perhaps the entire torso; some individuals feel the flush right to their toes. It is not an allergic reaction but simply an expected reaction due to the therapeutic properties of the vitamin. The flush causes a redness of the skin, which is also accompanied by itching and heat sensations. In some rare circumstances, niacin can induce nausea, vomiting, light-headedness, and chills. Many of my CFS patients actually like the flush and find that their nervous system problems substantially improve when using niacin regularly.

I suggest that patients begin by taking 100 mg of niacin at bedtime for the first two weeks. Once patients become accustomed to niacin's properties, I have them take 100 mg at breakfast, lunch, dinner, and before bed. If there are no observable benefits after 2–4 weeks of use, I increase the dose to 250 mg four times daily. If this increase does not produce any benefit after two weeks of use, the vitamin should be discontinued.

Like riboflavin, niacin can be used to treat migraine headaches. The only difference is that niacin is helpful at the onset of a migraine and does not function like riboflavin in preventing them. In acute migraine headaches, some of the symptoms arise from constriction of blood vessels within the brain, causing the migraine aura, followed by headache due to vasodilation of blood vessels surrounding the brain.[13] Because niacin has the ability to dilate blood vessels, several favorable reports have shown that it probably reverses the blood vessel constriction within the brain, which consequently prevents the dilation of blood vessels surrounding the brain.[14] It can be very effective when used at the onset of a migraine headache. For patients with CFS, I recommend 100 mg at the onset of a migraine, with instructions to repeat this dose up to four times in a day, if necessary. This method has a fairly good ability to stop migraines from becoming full-blown and incapacitating.

Other Solutions

Some other solutions to consider include the herbal (botanical) medicines *Ginkgo biloba* extract and vinpocetine, as both positively influence blood flow throughout the body and to the brain. Licorice tea may also prove beneficial.

Ginkgo Biloba Extract (GBE)

Ginkgo has demonstrated clinical efficacy for conditions characterized by cognitive impairment and for peripheral vascular disease (compromised blood flow to the periphery of the body).[15] It increases blood flow to the brain, positively influences brain chemicals known as neurotransmitters, and even protects the brain from injury.[16] A therapeutic trial of ginkgo should be considered because its active ingredients (flavonoids and terpenoids) have biological properties that positively influence the ANS and CNS and would potentially reverse the nervous system impairments that many people with CFS experience.

Start with a daily dose of GBE in the range of 60–240 mg; the extract should be standardized to 24 percent flavone glycosides and 6 percent terpene lactones. Side effects with GBE are rare, but some of my patients have reported rashes, nausea, and dizziness that cease once it is discontinued. For people with CFS who are also on blood-thinning medications, the use of ginkgo must be closely monitored by an experienced clinician. GBE was implicated in a case of bleeding within the brain in a patient taking a blood-thinner.[17]

Vinpocetine

Vinpocetine is an extract from the periwinkle plant, *Vinca minor*. This herb has clinically benefited patients with ischemic cerebrovascular disorders by reducing blood stickiness (viscosity).[18] These disorders are characterized by poor brain blood flow and cognitive impairment, which are similar to the nervous system impairments that CFS sufferers experience. Vinpocetine has also been useful as a treatment for degenerative senile cerebral dysfunction, demonstrating therapeutic effects upon cognitive and motor functions.[19] Vinpocetine improves blood flow and therefore the delivery of oxygen and nutrients to the organs and tissues of the body, particularly the brain.

The typical dose of vinpocetine is 10 mg three times daily. Side effects are rare, although a few of my patients have reported nausea and dizziness that disappear once the herbal agent is discontinued. Because it also possesses blood-thinning properties, the use of vinpocetine with blood-thinning medication needs to be closely supervised by an experienced clinician.

Licorice Tea

One of the potential benefits of licorice is that it can increase blood pressure and thus prevent the ANS disturbances that result from standing for prolonged periods of time or from shifting from a sitting to a standing position. Because of licorice's therapeutic properties, it should never be recommended to anyone with chronic fatigue who also has high blood pressure. As the majority of people with CFS have low blood pressure, licorice is potentially very useful.

Licorice increases cortisol, a hormone that can sometimes be low in chronic fatigue. A low cortisol level is thought to be implicated in the genesis of chronic fatigue.[20] A report in 1995 by a physician with CFS highlighted the therapeutic benefits of using licorice.[21] This physician had been unsuccessful in treating his CFS for around twenty months, but within several days of using licorice therapeutically he noticed a return of his previous physical and mental stamina.

Because depression and CFS can sometimes be clinically indistinguishable from each other, it is important to consider a 24-hour urinary free cortisol test prior to using licorice. If the cortisol level is high, the diagnosis is probably not chronic fatigue and is more likely to be depression.[22] If the cortisol level is low, the diagnosis is more likely to be CFS and it would be appropriate to consider licorice. However, a cortisol test is not always necessary because depression is not associated with enlarged lymph nodes, sore throat, and fever, so anyone with chronic fatigue who has these defining clinical features can try licorice.

Licorice tea can be purchased from any health food or grocery store. I have CFS patients drink 2–3 cups (16–24 ounces) per day. A quarter teaspoon of honey or lemon can be added to make the tea more palatable. Water retention and high blood pressure are rare side effects from licorice treatment, especially when it is administered as a tea. To reduce the potential of developing side effects, it is wise to eat high-potassium foods, such as bananas, honeydew melon, kiwis, lima beans, avocado, cantaloupe, oranges, and orange juice, when using licorice. People with CFS should not, however, consume any foods from this list if they are known to cause allergenic reactions.

TREATMENTS FOR OPTIMIZING AUTONOMIC AND CENTRAL NERVOUS SYSTEM FUNCTION

OLIGOANTIGENIC (ELIMINATION) DIET

THERAPEUTIC EFFECT: To identify and reduce dietary intolerances (food allergies)

DAILY DOSAGE: Follow a diet that does not contain implicated dietary items, or a rotation diet in which the foods are ingested infrequently

B-COMPLEX 50 OR 100

THERAPEUTIC EFFECT: Correction of deficiencies and improvement in memory and concentration

DAILY DOSAGE: One B-complex 50 or 100 with a meal (dose may be doubled if no apparent changes in cognitive symptoms after 4–8 weeks of use)

RIBOFLAVIN

THERAPEUTIC EFFECT: Prevention of migraine headaches

DAILY DOSAGE: 400 mg

NADH

THERAPEUTIC EFFECT: Correction of vitamin B_3 dependency and improvement in both the ANS and CNS impairments

DAILY DOSAGE: 10–20 mg

NIACIN

THERAPEUTIC EFFECT: Correction of vitamin B_3 dependency and increased blood flow throughout the body and brain

DAILY DOSAGE: 100 mg at bedtime, increasing the amount slowly over time to 100 mg four times daily (some people might need 250 mg four times daily)

THERAPEUTIC EFFECT: Can stop (abort) acute migraine headaches by vasodilating the blood vessels within the brain

DAILY DOSAGE: 100 mg at the onset of a migraine; can repeat this dose up to four times, if necessary

***GINKGO BILOBA* EXTRACT**

THERAPEUTIC EFFECT: Increases blood flow to the brain, positively influences neurotransmitters, and protects the brain from injury

DAILY DOSAGE: 60–240 mg

VINPOCETINE

THERAPEUTIC EFFECT: Improves blood flow and therefore the delivery of oxygen and nutrients to the organs and tissues of the body, particularly the brain

DAILY DOSAGE: 10 mg three times daily

LICORICE TEA

THERAPEUTIC EFFECT: Improves blood flow to the brain, increases blood pressure, raises cortisol levels, and helps to moderate symptoms of ANS disturbances

DAILY DOSAGE: 2–3 cups (16–24 ounces)

Summary

Many people with chronic fatigue experience autonomic and central nervous system symptoms that lead to light-headedness, fatigue when standing, and cognitive deficits involving memory and concentration. Supplementing with a daily B-complex 50 or

100 vitamin is essential, as those with CFS might be deficient in several B vitamins (particularly thiamine, riboflavin, and pyridoxine). These vitamins can be used therapeutically to improve memory and concentration. Additional riboflavin might be needed in CFS cases with migraines. The use of various forms of vitamin B_3 might be particularly helpful since the nervous system complications of a B_3 dependency mimic the ANS and CNS system problems that people with CFS experience. The coenzyme of B_3, NADH, has been shown in clinical studies to benefit those with chronic fatigue. The niacin form of B_3 possesses biochemical properties that also support the nervous system. Niacin improves blood flow throughout the body, and likely the brain as well, by inducing vasodilation of blood vessels. For those with migraines, niacin has been shown to stop acute migraine attacks from progressing.

Three herbal medications—*Ginkgo biloba* extract, vinpocetine, and licorice tea—increase blood flow to the brain. Ginkgo and vinpocetine can reduce symptoms of cognitive impairment, while licorice helps to increase blood pressure and normalize the autonomic disturbances that are common among people with chronic fatigue.

CHAPTER 5

A DETOXIFICATION PROGRAM FOR CHRONIC FATIGUE

Earlier in this book, research was presented about the relationship between toxic agents and chronic fatigue syndrome (CFS). It is well known that exposure to toxins can produce an illness that would be clinically indistinguishable from CFS. The most implicated toxins are the organochlorine and organophosphate chemicals that have widespread use in both domestic and industrial settings, in items such as insecticides and pesticides. People with CFS who believe they are toxic can usually recall an event or exposure that seemed to trigger the onset of their illness. They might have lived near a golf course, where the spraying of pesticides is common practice, or perhaps they grew up on a farm where chemicals were needed to spare the crops from pest destruction. Some may believe that environmental toxic exposures created their illness, and they are probably correct, since they can pinpoint the exact time and place when the exposures occurred and when their symptoms began.

For environmentally toxic CFS sufferers, a detoxification program should be instituted immediately so that fat-soluble toxins can be safely and effectively eliminated from the body. Detoxification is the body's ability to transform a fat-soluble compound into a water-soluble compound so that it can be eliminated.[1] Although the urinary route of excretion actively removes transformed fat-soluble compounds, it is not always an effective avenue of elimination. Fat-soluble toxins can persist for years or even decades because they were never effectively removed from the body. People with chronic fatigue can have excessive amounts of fat-soluble organochlorine and organophosphate compounds that continue to wreak havoc since they remain imbedded in tissues, particularly fat, and in organs such as the liver, kidneys, and even the brain.[2]

When this occurs, other avenues of elimination must be encouraged—respiration or breathing, sweating through the skin, and increasing the bulk and frequency of bowel movements—so that toxins can be successfully purged from the body. To achieve this, a detoxification program encompassing diet, vitamins, exercise, infrared sauna therapy, and other treatments is necessary. Numerous studies have documented the clinical effectiveness of a detoxification program for CFS that includes these elements.[3]

Dietary Solutions

As a first step in detoxifying, people with chronic fatigue should consider following an oligoantigenic (elimination) diet, followed by a challenge phase to pinpoint dietary intolerances (food allergies). Once all implicated dietary items have been identified, they should be strictly avoided or ingested only once every four days to limit ongoing allergic reactions. This is vital to eliminating toxins due to environmental exposures. A cleaner diet reduces the intake of diet-derived organochlorine and organophosphate compounds and diminishes any ongoing damage that might result from a poor diet.

Cleaner and less allergenic diets are normally much higher in fiber than diets that are allergenic, which often include processed and refined foods. When fiber intake is sufficient, the fiber binds intestinal toxins and encourages their elimination through the bowels.[4] Each day, the liver makes bile and dumps it into the intestines, where its toxic load can be absorbed by fiber and excreted as part of the stool. When the diet has an insufficient amount of fiber, the result is inadequate binding and an increase in the amount of toxins that find their way back into the bloodstream (reabsorption).

Certain foods should also be added to a cleaner diet, as they can improve the body's resistance to toxic exposures and support its ability to eliminate toxins. The most important foods to include are vegetables of the *Brassica* family and citrus fruits. Foods of the *Brassica* family include cabbage, broccoli, cauliflower, and Brussels sprouts. They contain health-promoting chemicals that support the liver's ability to detoxify toxins and that protect against the development of cancer.[5] These vegetables should be washed thoroughly and then steamed or boiled; they should not be eaten raw, as people with CFS often find raw vegetables difficult to digest. As for how much to consume, I encourage two to four servings each day (about one-half to one cup of any vegetable usually constitutes a single serving).

Citrus fruits, such as oranges and tangerines, should also be consumed as long as they do not themselves produce allergic manifestations. (Any allergies should have been identified while doing the oligoantigenic diet.) These citrus fruits contain a compound known as limonene that induces detoxification enzymes within the liver and even neutralizes cancer-causing toxins.[6] For the purposes of supporting detoxification, two to four servings daily should be consumed (one serving is equivalent to approximately one orange or one medium-sized tangerine).

Vitamin Solutions

Vitamin B_3 (Niacin)

The long-term effects from using therapeutic doses of niacin are reductions in both cardiovascular risk and disease. Niacin achieves this beneficial effect because it reduces the mobilization (release) of fatty acids and favorably alters the cholesterol profile.[7] Fatty acids are acids produced when fats are broken down. For the purposes of detoxification, niacin is used only on the days when undergoing infrared sauna therapy. When used this way, the initial reduction in mobilized fatty acids from taking niacin is followed by a short-lived increase in the release of fatty acids[8], facilitating the removal of fat-stored toxins through the skin.

Begin by taking 100 mg of niacin immediately before your first infrared sauna treatment and the same amount immediately afterward. Once you become accustomed to niacin's properties, increase to 250 mg immediately before and after sauna treatments. Studies using niacin as part of a detoxification program rely on much higher dosages, but because people with CFS can be very sensitive, it is best not to increase the niacin unless there is proper medical supervision. The possible side effects from using niacin have already been discussed (see Chapter 4).

Multiple Vitamin Supplement

A multiple vitamin typically contains vitamins A, C, D, E, and all the B-complex vitamins, including folic acid. People undergoing detoxification need to include a multiple vitamin for several important reasons. Because sweating is dramatically increased, more vitamins will be lost through the sweat, which can potentially create deficiencies. It is important to replace these loses with a multiple vitamin. Going through a detoxification program also speeds up the body's metabolism, so more vitamins are needed to keep pace with the increased metabolic demands. A multiple vitamin also helps the body handle the additional detoxification demands that result when fat-stored toxins are mobilized from the various tissues and organs.

Only use a multiple vitamin that is free of common allergens and is in a vegetarian-based capsule or tablet, which makes it easier to digest. While undergoing detoxification, it is best to take a multiple vitamin with each main meal, and sometimes with snacks as well. This level is much more than what the label typically recommends but is needed to compensate for the losses and additional metabolic demands of detoxification. Side effects from multiple vitamins are extremely rare, but could include nausea or vomiting when taken on an empty stomach.

A multiple vitamin also helps to fill in gaps caused by diets lacking in micronutrients. I wish that we were able to obtain all of our required nutrients from diet alone. The problem is that our diets have diverged considerably from what our ancestors used to eat over 40,000 years ago. We consumed a much more nutrient-dense diet with optimal quantities of antioxidant vitamins, healthy fats, and other essential nutrients; a diet that was specific to the needs of our genetic make-up.[9] Our genes have not changed much, but our diets have. Through over-processing, poor soil conditions, and long-distance shipping, our food has become nutrient-deficient. This has contributed to the increase in the development of chronic diseases such as cancer, heart disease, diabetes, and obesity.[10] For these simple and important reasons, it is paramount that everyone regularly take a multiple vitamin supplement.

Other Solutions

Exercise

Exercise aids the detoxification process by promoting both the circulation of blood to the tissues[11] and the release of fat.[12] By facilitating the release of fat, exercise presumably increases the release of fat-stored toxins as well.[13] For optimal detoxification results, perform low-intensity aerobic exercise (for example, brisk walking) for 10–20 minutes immediately before infrared sauna therapy.

I recommend that people with chronic fatigue adopt a regular exercise program. To be effective, it need not lead to more muscle microtrauma, pain, and injury. A regular exercise program should ideally lead to more self-reliance and autonomy, and the intensity level should always remain low. It is difficult to be specific about how long the exercise session should last. You need to slowly increase your exercise tolerance and duration over a prolonged period of time.

Prior to engaging in an exercise program, you must receive a thorough evaluation. This should include assessing the appropriateness of the exercise program, cardiovascular function and risk factors, joint function and the presence of osteoarthritis, muscle function, medication use, concomitant problems that might reduce the effectiveness or usefulness of exercise, and the current level of physical fitness.

Infrared Sauna

An infrared sauna uses ceramic heaters to produce radiant heat (thermal energy), an invisible form of energy that heats objects directly.[14] It facilitates the excretion of fatty acids through the skin, and thus increases the elimination of fat-soluble toxins.[15] Infrared sauna therapy is able to produce a greater amount of sweat than steam saunas because the temperatures do not have to be nearly as high, usually in the range of 45–50° Celsius or 113–122° Fahrenheit.[16] Individuals sweat more in infrared saunas because they can remain in them for longer periods of time.

Two studies have evaluated the therapeutic effects of infrared sauna therapy on patients with chronic fatigue. In one study, two patients received infrared sauna therapy at 60°C (140°F) once daily for a total of thirty-five sessions.[17] Then, each patient returned once or twice each week as an outpatient for one year. After 15–25 outpatient sessions, symptoms such as fatigue, pain, sleep disturbances, and low-grade fever dramatically improved. They experienced no relapse or exacerbation of symptoms during the year on outpatient therapy. Another study demonstrated that infrared sauna dramatically improved symptoms such as fatigue, pain, and low-grade fever, in two patients with CFS; eleven others from the same study also showed improvements in fatigue and pain.[18]

People with chronic fatigue should use an infrared sauna daily, if possible, for the first month of treatment; usually between the fifteenth and twenty-fifth treatments, symptom reduction becomes apparent. The temperature during the first few treatments should be on the low side, somewhere around 45°C (113°F). After several treatments, the temperature can be gradually increased to 60°C (140°F). Treatment duration is dependent on your ability to withstand the heat and to not suffer any relapses. During the first few sessions, limit the treatment duration to about 15–20 minutes; eventually, you will be capable of sixty minutes of sauna therapy, which is desirable.

During infrared sauna therapy, you should drink as much water as you need and should take electrolyte replacement drinks as well. There are now a number of natural electrolyte replacement drinks that do not contain artificial colors and chemicals and that have sufficient amounts of salt (sodium), potassium, and other minerals to help offset the losses that result from sweating. This also protects against heat exhaustion (characterized by heavy sweating, paleness, muscle cramps, tiredness, weakness, dizziness, headache, nausea or vomiting, and fainting), which usually develops after several days of heat exposure.

People with CFS should not be treated with infrared sauna therapy if they have severe lymphedema (limb swelling), are pregnant or breastfeeding, or have a pacemaker or metal implant.[19] Chronic fatigue sufferers who also have kidney, heart, or liver disease, hypoglycemia, or seizure disorders can be treated with infrared sauna, but must be closely monitored.[20]

Multiple Mineral Supplement

Like the vitamin supplement, a multiple mineral supplement is also needed due to the losses that result from sweating and from the increased metabolic and detoxification demands placed on the body. A multiple mineral usually contains calcium, magnesium, zinc, selenium, copper, chromium, potassium, and sometimes manganese and molybdenum. There is no need to use a multiple mineral that contains iron, as the dose would not be therapeutic even for people with CFS who are iron-deficient. The supplement should be free of common allergens and in a vegetarian-based capsule or tablet. The multiple mineral should not be taken with meals but rather before and after sauna therapy. So, if the recommended daily dose is two capsules, then take one immediately before and another immediately after the infrared sauna therapy. There should be no side effects from taking a multiple mineral supplement.

Polyunsaturated Oils (Fats)

Each day, the liver manufactures bile, which serves as a carrier of toxins that get dumped into the intestines. While in the intestines, some of the toxins can get absorbed by fiber and passed with the stool, while the remaining toxins will simply get reabsorbed into the bloodstream, where they can continue to create problems. A therapeutic amount of polyunsaturated oils can either block the toxins from getting reabsorbed into the bloodstream or they can facilitate the excretion of toxins with the stool.[21] When fat-stored toxins are mobilized as a result of the detoxification process, supplemental polyunsaturated oils will replace the fats that were released from adipose tissues.[22] These polyunsaturated oils thus alter the content of fat tissue that was previously laden with environmental toxins.

A good source of polyunsaturated oils is the omega-3, omega-6, and omega-9 varieties:

- Omega-3: Alpha-linolenic acid, eicosapentaenoic acid (EPA), docosahexaenoic acid (DHA)
- Omega-6: Linoleic acid, gamma-linolenic acid, dihomo-gamma linolenic acid, arachidonic acid
- Omega-9: Oleic acid

These are termed *essential fatty acids* because the body must receive a sufficient daily amount from diet or supplementation; otherwise, deficiencies of them can lead to problems with detoxification as well as other physiological impairments.

Polyunsaturated oils should be taken in a softgel pill, which limits oxidation and rancidity. Many supplements containing the three types of oil are available, with each softgel providing approximately 1,200 mg of polyunsaturated oils. When undergoing a detoxification program, two softgels (2,400 mg) should be taken with each main meal of the day. No side effects should occur, but supplementing with these polyunsaturated oils can rarely cause loose stools or diarrhea.

Glutathione

When undergoing a detoxification program, more chemicals get filtered through the liver because they become released from fat tissues and organs. One of the most important nutrients that the body needs for healthy detoxification is the tripeptide glutathione, also known as reduced L-glutathione (GSH). Supplemental GSH helps to maintain glutathione levels within the red blood cells of the body and it is also needed by the liver to help with detoxification. The liver is the main organ involved in detoxifying chemicals, and it requires sufficient amounts of glutathione to neutralize toxins and make them more easily excreted in the urine or bile.[23]

The typical therapeutic dose of GSH is 1.0–1.5 teaspoons per day, providing approximately 420–600 mg. Over-the-counter liposomal (phospholipid-derived) GSH preparations appear to be the most effective form for raising red blood cell and liver levels of glutathione. I am not aware of any side effects from the use of liposomal GSH.

DETOXIFICATION PROGRAM FOR CFS

OLIGOANTIGENIC (ELIMINATION) DIET

THERAPEUTIC EFFECT: To identify and reduce dietary intolerances (food allergies)

DAILY DOSAGE: Follow a diet that does not contain any implicated dietary items, or a rotation diet in which the foods are ingested infrequently

BRASSICA VEGETABLES AND CITRUS FRUITS

THERAPEUTIC EFFECT: Support the liver's ability to detoxify and protect against cancer

DAILY DOSAGE: 2–4 servings of foods from each group

NIACIN

THERAPEUTIC EFFECT: Facilitates the removal of fat-stored toxins through the skin

DAILY DOSAGE: 100–250 mg immediately before and after infrared sauna treatment

MULTIPLE VITAMIN

THERAPEUTIC EFFECT: For replenishing nutrient losses from sweating and from increased metabolic and detoxification demands on the body

DAILY DOSAGE: Take a multiple vitamin with each main meal, and sometimes with snacks as well

EXERCISE (PREFERABLY AEROBIC)

THERAPEUTIC EFFECT: Aids detoxification by promoting blood circulation and the release of fat

DAILY DOSAGE: Slowly increase duration 10–20 minutes immediately before infrared sauna therapy

INFRARED SAUNA

THERAPEUTIC EFFECT: Facilitates the excretion of fatty acids through the skin, increasing the elimination of fat-soluble toxins

DAILY DOSAGE: Duration should be limited to 15–20 minutes for the first few sessions; can be increased to 60 minutes once you develop tolerance

MULTIPLE MINERAL

THERAPEUTIC EFFECT: For replenishing nutrient losses from sweating and from increased metabolic and detoxification demands on the body

DAILY DOSAGE: Take the recommended dose, half immediately before and half immediately after the infrared sauna session

POLYUNSATURATED OILS (OMEGA-3, OMEGA-6, AND OMEGA-9)

THERAPEUTIC EFFECT: Block toxins from getting reabsorbed into the bloodstream and facilitate the excretion of toxins

DAILY DOSAGE: Two softgels (2,400 mg) should be taken with each main meal of the day

GLUTATHIONE

THERAPEUTIC EFFECT: Maintains glutathione levels within red blood cells and supports the liver's detoxification pathways

DAILY DOSAGE: 1.0–1.5 teaspoons of liposomal GSH, providing approximately 420–600 mg

Summary

Some people with chronic fatigue suffer from environmental toxicities, usually the result of exposures to organochlorine and organophosphate chemicals. These toxic chemicals remain embedded in fat tissues and organs of the body, such as the liver, kidneys, and brain. The symptoms produced by exposures to these toxins are clinically indistinguishable from those that typify CFS.

A detoxification program should be instituted so that these toxins can be eliminated from the body. A program that relies on diet, exercise, infrared sauna, vitamins, and other treatments has been scientifically validated. For those with CFS to effectively eliminate toxins, they need to adopt a detoxification program that uses a combination of these treatments in a medically supervised setting.

CHAPTER 6

RESTORING BALANCE TO THE IMMUNE SYSTEM

Poor nutritional habits (such as eating too much junk food and sugar) or having specific nutrient deficiencies (vitamin A, vitamin C, and zinc) will impair the immune system, making us more susceptible to infections. When immune status has been compromised by poor nutrition, the infections we actually succumb to become much more virulent and damaging. This is perhaps one of the central reasons why so many individuals that develop chronic fatigue syndrome (CFS) have an immune system that is chronically over-activated.

Not only are people with CFS vulnerable to the deleterious effects of a triggering agent like a virus, but it is highly probable that a virus or some other infectious agent causes more significant immune system damage as a consequence of inadequate nutrition. This is a vicious cycle: inadequate nutrition increased the vulnerability to infection, and once the infection triggered the immune system, inadequate nutritional status allowed the infection to persist longer, leading to a state of chronic immune system activation and the eventual development of CFS. Key symptoms of immune system dysfunction among CFS sufferers include: general malaise; being chronically fatigued; having a chronic sore throat or sinus congestion; experiencing daily muscle aches and pains; and potentially having abnormal skin, hair, and nail changes.

To restore balance to the immune system, it is essential that people with CFS change their daily nutritional habits, which must include a cleaner and healthier diet and supplementation with vitamins and other nutrients.

Dietary Solutions

Dietary modifications can have a significant positive impact on the immune system. We have already addressed the need to include an oligoantigenic (elimination) diet as a method of identifying dietary intolerances (food allergies)—foods that need to be avoided or ingested infrequently (see Chapter 3). This helps to maximize the functioning of the immune system. Dietary intolerance is a major underlying factor among individuals with recurrent infections, due to irritation and inflammation of various tissues.[1] Since inflamed and irritated respiratory passages increase susceptibility to infection, the elimination of food allergies can reduce the incidence of recurrent colds, bronchitis, yeast infections, and even herpes simplex outbreaks.

Those with CFS need to reduce their chances of getting upper respiratory infections or other types of infections, since any infection will cause a flare-up in their condition. Eliminating dietary intolerances helps to maintain the health of the immune system and also reduces the frequency of infections—this inevitably improves quality of life among CFS sufferers.

Eliminate Simple Carbohydrates

Simple carbohydrates are sweeteners found in foods such as pastries, cakes, and candy. Some common examples are glucose, sucrose, and lactose. In a study involving healthy adults, drinking 24 ounces of a cola beverage delayed the ability of white blood cells to effectively eliminate bacteria by 50 percent within forty-five minutes.[2] In another study, adults who ingested 100 grams of carbohydrate (from glucose, fructose, sucrose, honey, or orange juice) showed a significantly decreased ability of specialized immune cells to engulf bacteria compared to fasting values.[3] The impairment lasted 1–2 hours after ingesting the carbohydrate drink and even remained abnormal when measured five hours later. If you have chronic fatigue, you should restrict your consumption of simple carbohydrates, otherwise you will be more susceptible to infection.

Eliminate Caffeine

Caffeine and its major metabolite, paraxanthine, suppress several immune system functions:

- The ability for specialized white blood cells to migrate to areas where they are needed
- The production of the beneficial immune system compound tumor necrosis factor-alpha (TNF-alpha)
- The activity of lymphocytes, specialized cells that help to fight viruses and stimulate protective antibodies[4]

People with chronic fatigue should eliminate caffeine from their diet.

Eat Adequate Protein

Protein intake should not be reduced or avoided when trying to improve the health of the immune system. People with chronic fatigue are particularly prone to the negative effects of not eating enough protein, and some might even develop a severe form of malnutrition called protein-energy malnutrition, in which their protein and energy intakes have been very poor for prolonged periods of time. CFS sufferers might also experience other medical issues that prevent adequate intakes of protein, which would also compromise their immune system. The immunological consequences of inadequate protein include problems in fighting viruses, engulfing bacteria, and in the production of antibodies.[5]

Increasing the daily intake of protein might be an effective strategy to improve immune function in people with CFS whose intakes are inadequate. An acceptable daily intake of protein is 0.75–0.80 grams per kilogram of body weight, although more than 1.0 g/kg of body weight might be necessary when muscle mass has dramatically declined. For example, a 130-pound woman would need approximately 47 grams of protein daily to ensure an adequate intake:

130 pounds ÷ 2.2 = 59.09 kg (convert pounds to kilograms)
59.09 kg × 0.80 g = 47.27 grams of protein

As long as they do not cause adverse (allergic) reactions, the following foods are good sources of protein: wild cold-water fish (salmon, mackerel, sardines, and herring), white meat poultry (without the skin), yogurt, eggs, beans, soy, pork, and lean beef.

Vitamin Solutions

Vitamin A

Vitamin A (retinol) is one of the most critical nutrients for maintaining a healthy immune system. It plays a vital role in the development and differentiation of infection-fighting white blood cells as well as other cells of the immune system.[6] According to many studies, vitamin A has a major role in preventing morbidity and death from infectious diseases, including reduction in deaths from diarrheal disease (39 percent), from respiratory diseases (70 percent), and from other causes of death (34 percent).[7]

I recommend that all patients with CFS supplement with 5,000–20,000 IU of vitamin A each day to prevent infections.[8] Since the flu can cause major flare-ups of CFS, I sometimes recommend that my patients take 100,000 IU of vitamin A at the onset of their flu symptoms and another 100,000 IU at bedtime.[9] Patients usually feel better the next morning when taking these optimal doses. Sometimes this strategy fails and patients then need to take 100,000 IU twice daily for seven days to eradicate the influenza infection.[10] In light of vitamin A's ability to cause birth defects, pregnant women or women wishing to become pregnant should never take more than 5,000 IU of vitamin A each day.

Vitamin C

Vitamin C is perhaps the most important water-soluble antioxidant in the body. It works synergistically with other antioxidants, especially vitamin E, where it helps to regenerate pre-oxidized forms of the vitamin.[11] Vitamin C is needed in the production of interferon, an important stimulator of the immune system. It also improves the ability of white blood cells to fight infections and stimulates immune cells to attack other cells infected with a virus or that are cancerous.[12] In a small study involving eight healthy men, vitamin C deficiency led to decreased blood levels of glutathione and vitamin B_3 coenzymes (antioxidants), a more than 50 percent decline in blood levels and white blood cell levels of vitamin C, and delayed immune system responsiveness.[13]

While an experimental deficiency of vitamin C increases susceptibility to infection, the results of human studies using high dosages to prevent and treat infections have been more equivocal. Nevertheless, there are important benefits from supplementing with vitamin C. In a published review of vitamin C and the common cold, a dosage of 1–6 grams per day decreased the duration of the common cold by almost a full day (or 20 percent).[14] In another review, it was determined that taking large supplemental doses is not justified, except among individuals exposed to brief periods of severe physical exercise or extreme cold environments, where there might be tremendous benefit from supplementation.[15] When using vitamin C to prevent and treat pneumonia, a review concluded that the effects were too weak to recommend its routine use at the present time.[16]

However, I strongly disagree with these conclusions. The published scientific papers of vitamin C pioneer Robert F. Cathcart, M.D., prove that vitamin C is effective for treating numerous infections. Unfortunately, his work has been virtually ignored by mainstream medicine. Dr. Cathcart described the usefulness of huge amounts of vitamin C on a daily basis when faced with a severe infection like pneumonia[17], because the stress of infection increases the body's need for the vitamin. He reported that more than 100 grams (100,000 mg) of vitamin C was needed orally to assist the body in recovering from pneumonia.

People with chronic fatigue are unusually susceptible to infections, such as the common cold and even pneumonia, and are always under more biochemical and physiological stress than individuals without CFS. Vitamin C is a relatively benign vitamin, and there might be considerable value for CFS sufferers to take it daily as prophylaxis and to increase their daily amounts should a common cold or pneumonia develop. The therapeutic benefits from high-dose vitamin C supplementation might prove significantly more substantial than the conclusions derived from published studies in mainstream medical journals.

For prevention, I usually recommend 2,000–6,000 mg daily of vitamin C. When being used to treat a cold or in conjunction with medications to treat pneumonia, the daily amount should be increased to an amount just below bowel tolerance. To determine the bowel tolerance amount, I recommend that my patients take 1,000–4,000 mg of vitamin C every hour until they experience lots of gas or have diarrhea (neither of which are dangerous). If, for example, these nuisance effects occur at 12,000 mg, then bowel tolerance has been achieved. A vitamin C dose 500–1,000 mg below bowel tolerance is recommended.

The body needs lots of vitamin C when under the stresses of an infection, and the bowel tolerance doses of vitamin C can be much higher than the amount cited here. It is well established that the more ill a person is, the more vitamin C they will need and be able to tolerate before experiencing symptoms of bowel tolerance.[18] The daily amount of vitamin C can then be lowered as a cold or pneumonia improves and the body recovers. It is important that you learn how to figure this out and make the necessary adjustments on your own.

A few years ago, I had a terrible cold and my bowel tolerance limit was around 25,000 mg for several days. As I improved, I substantially reduced my daily amount to around 7,000 mg. To this day, I continue to require around 7,000–9,000 mg of vitamin C daily to maintain good health. Any more than this amount typically produces symptoms of bowel tolerance, unless my requirements change, such as when I am under severe stress or have an infection.

Vitamin E

Vitamin E is an important fat-soluble antioxidant that protects fats within cell membranes from oxidative damage.[19] Deficiency of vitamin E results in a significantly weakened immune system.[20] One study demonstrated that taking varying dosages of vitamin E for four months improved certain parameters of immunity in healthy elderly subjects.[21] In those taking 200 mg each day, there was a 65 percent increase in immune system responsiveness and a sixfold increase in the production of antibodies in response to both hepatitis B and tetanus vaccinations. In another study, elderly nursing home residents were administered 200 IU of vitamin E for one year to determine its effect on respiratory tract infections.[22] Vitamin E was able to reduce the incidence of the common cold but did not influence lower respiratory tract infections.

It is difficult to apply these findings directly to people with chronic fatigue since elderly populations were studied and the dosages of vitamin E varied; also, the form of vitamin E used tended to be synthetic. The dosage with the most optimal effects appears to be a minimum of 200 mg each day. The natural form of vitamin E (D-alpha tocopherol) should be used rather than the less effective synthetic form (D,L-alpha tocopherol). It is clear that vitamin E improves certain parameters of the immune system, particularly augmenting the antibody response and reducing upper respiratory infections. People with CFS are always at risk of getting infections, especially colds, and should derive benefit from vitamin E supplementation.

All those with chronic fatigue should supplement with at least 200 mg (approximately 300 IU) of natural vitamin E. Higher dosages (500 mg or approximately 750 IU) might be needed to yield greater therapeutic benefits at balancing the immune system and reducing the incidence of upper respiratory infections.

Vitamin B_6

Vitamin B_6 (pyridoxine) is critical to the functioning of immune system cells, especially since they are all rapidly dividing cells.[23] It also assists in the production of glutathione, a major antioxidant in the body that plays an important role in the lymphocytes that respond to viral infections and cancer.[24] A deficiency of B_6 negatively affects the development of lymphocytes, reduces immune system responsiveness, and weakens the production of infection-fighting antibodies.[25]

While the majority of studies that demonstrate immunological benefits from vitamin B_6 supplementation involve patients with compromised immunity[26], chronic fatigue sufferers also have compromised immune function and would thus benefit from daily supplementation. An effective therapeutic dose of vitamin B_6 is 50–100 mg each day, but some people might require higher daily doses, such as 250 mg. There should be no side effects from taking these specified amounts of vitamin B_6, even though there have been some controversial reports of peripheral or sensory neuropathy (numbness and tingling in the arms and legs) and even central nervous system toxicity from taking supplemental pyridoxine.

In over ten years of clinical practice, I have not observed any toxic side effects from the use of vitamin B_6 and have prescribed higher daily dosages (even a few thousand milligrams) of pyridoxine to numerous patients. My clinical experiences are in line with evidence reported by renowned nutritional expert Alan R. Gaby, M.D.[27] He highlights several key pieces of information that remove any toxicity concerns involving the doses that I have recommended:

- If we use animal studies to extrapolate a dose of vitamin B_6 that would cause neurotoxicity, it would be equivalent to 3,000 mg per day for a 60-kilogram (132-pound) person.
- The only reports of sensory neuropathy occurred when patients were taking 2,000 mg or more of pyridoxine each day, although some patients reported toxicity from only 500 mg daily.
- One report involved a patient taking only 200 mg, but the reliability of this particular case has been challenged.

A retrospective study assessed toxicity from vitamin B_6 and found that supplementation with doses ranging from 30–230 mg daily was associated with decreases in symptoms of sensory neuropathy among individuals who had these symptoms prior to taking the vitamin.[28] The use of supplemental pyridoxine was also associated with reductions in insomnia, rash, and acne. These published sources of evidence lead me to believe that there is virtually no chance of developing any toxicity symptoms from 50–100 mg of vitamin B_6 each day and almost no concerns from taking 250 mg daily.

Other Solutions

Polyunsaturated Oils (Fats)

Omega-3 essential fatty acids are polyunsaturated oils that must be obtained from the diet or supplementation since the body needs them to function optimally (hence, the term *essential*). The omega-3 oils contain an important immune-modulating component known as eicosapentaenoic acid (EPA). When the diet contains regular amounts of omega-3 essential fatty acids, the EPA component partially replaces another type of oil, known as arachidonic acid, within the membranes of the body's cells. Since arachidonic acid increases the production of inflammatory compounds, the partial replacement by EPA will help decrease inflammation.[29]

High-dose omega-3 supplementation is required when immune-modulating effects are sought after, but these benefits have been limited to diseases (such as rheumatoid arthritis and inflammatory bowel disease) that are associated with severe immune dysfunction. It is unlikely that increasing omega-3s will produce any marked immune system changes when administered to healthy subjects.

Studies have shown a need for these oils among people with chronic fatigue because they do not adequately produce EPA from dietary precursors, such as flaxseed oil. There is some impairment in the body's ability to produce enough EPA, which is the result of a defective enzyme.[30] There is even data showing that an insufficient amount of dietary omega-3s might play a role in causing CFS, including specific immunological defects.[31] A review published in 2006 concluded that high intakes of omega-3 oils had marked immune-modulating effects by decreasing the production of inflammatory compounds and free radicals.[32]

To derive immunological benefits from omega-3 oils, people

with CFS should take a minimum of 2,400 mg of EPA each day. With any omega-3 oil, it is possible to experience gastrointestinal side effects, such as gas, burping, and bloating. To reduce the occurrence of these side effects, I suggest an enteric-coated omega-3 capsule, so that digestion primarily occurs in the small intestine instead of the stomach. Another option is to try liquid preparations of omega-3 oils, which are associated with very few, if any, gastrointestinal side effects.

Zinc

The mineral zinc is of critical importance to the ongoing health of the immune system. It is a cofactor for deoxyribonucleic acid (DNA) and ribonucleic acid (RNA) enzymes as well as for the important antioxidant enzyme superoxide dismutase (SOD). Recall that DNA contains our genetic material and RNA enables the body to produce protein. Zinc is also an essential nutrient for all immune cells, particularly cells that are involved in fighting infections.[33]

Zinc deficiency is characterized by many immune system derangements that reduce the body's ability to fight infections.[34] A deficiency of the mineral is associated with diseases such as malabsorption syndrome, chronic liver disease, chronic kidney disease, sickle cell anemia, diabetes, and malignancy.[35] In one study, fifty healthy elderly subjects were given elemental zinc (45 mg per day) or placebo for twelve months.[36] The zinc-supplemented group had a significantly reduced incidence of infections, higher blood levels of zinc, and markers of oxidative damage were lower. Elderly people, children, and adolescents undergoing rapid growth spurts are more vulnerable to zinc deficiency, but I would include chronic fatigue sufferers as well. Many individuals with CFS tend to have limited diets, which increases their risk of developing zinc deficiency. Additionally, zinc should be used as a treatment to prevent the common cold, which might help to reduce exacerbations of CFS triggered by cold viruses.

The daily therapeutic dose of zinc should be 50 mg of elemental zinc, but this amount can be increased to 80 mg of elemental zinc if needed. Good types of zinc supplements are zinc amino acid chelate, zinc citrate, and zinc picolinate. Read the labels carefully when purchasing zinc supplements to determine how much elemental zinc is in the product; this is the dose that is important. When supplementing with zinc, people with CFS should also add 1–2 mg of copper each day to prevent complications from long-term zinc supplementation, such as a reduction in white blood cells.

Selenium

As an essential trace element, selenium plays a critical role in guarding against oxidative damage and regulating immune function.[37] Deficiency of selenium is characterized by a decreased ability to fight viral infections and increased damage by oxygen free radicals.[38] In a study involving twenty-two healthy adults with relatively low blood concentrations of selenium, subjects were given either selenium (50–100 micrograms each day) or placebo for fifteen weeks.[39] These modest supplemental doses produced favorable effects on their immune systems by increasing their ability to clear the poliovirus. The authors noted that these supplementary levels were below the amounts of selenium needed to fully optimize immune function. In an article discussing nutritional strategies for the elderly, various micronutrients were suggested as a way to reverse the immune dysfunction associated with aging.[40] Selenium, zinc, and vitamin E were recommended to address this problem and reduce the risk of infection. There is also an abundance of data supporting selenium (200 micrograms daily) as a treatment for serious diseases that are associated with marked immune dysfunction, such as human immunodeficiency virus infection or squamous cell carcinoma of the head and neck.[41]

Because selenium can markedly improve the immune system's response to fighting viral infections and even specific cancers, it makes sense to include this trace mineral in a plan targeted to restore immune function among those with CFS. High-selenium yeast is an organic source of the trace mineral and is preferable to other forms of selenium.[42] All CFS sufferers should supplement with 200 micrograms of high-selenium yeast. If higher doses are needed, this should not produce any concerns since there has been no toxicity from using high-selenium yeast in amounts as high as 800 micrograms daily.[43]

Plant Sterols

Plant sterols and sterolins are cholesterol-like molecules obtained from plants that contain beta-sitosterol (BSS), which is found in the serum and tissues of healthy individuals.[44] A derivative of BSS, beta-sitosterol glycoside (BSSG), is also found in the serum. A nutritional supplement that contains a mixture of both has been shown to have immune-balancing properties.[45] Test-tube experiments have demonstrated that the sterol mixture increases T-helper type 1 (T_h1) cells and inhibits or does not change T-helper type 2 (T_h2) cells. An overactive T_h1 is often linked to autoimmune diseases (such as multiple sclerosis), while an overactive T_h2 is linked to allergies.[46]

There is clinical evidence demonstrating a heightened T_h2 response and a dampened T_h1 response among those with chronic fatigue.[47] Immune dysfunction in CFS is characterized by a predominance of T_h2 pro-inflammatory cytokines, which is associated with physiological and psychological dysfunction and activation of latent viruses or other pathogens.[48] The use of the sterol mixture might have important clinical implications because an enhanced T_h1 response might facilitate the clearance of particular pathogens (such as cold and flu viruses) and would also correct immune abnormalities associated with CFS.

The sterol mixture should provide 20 mg of beta-sitosterol and 200 micrograms of beta-sitosterol glycoside per pill.[49] People with CFS should take two pills three times daily for the first month, followed by a maintenance dose of three pills thereafter. Take on an empty stomach at least one hour before meals; do not take it with animal fats and milk because absorption will be impaired.

RESTORING THE IMMUNE SYSTEM

DIETARY MODIFICATIONS

THERAPEUTIC EFFECT: Helps to maintain the health of the immune system and also reduces the frequency of infections

DAILY DOSAGE: Follow a diet that does not contain any dietary intolerances (food allergies), eliminate simple carbohydrates and caffeine, and consume an adequate amount of protein each day

VITAMIN A

THERAPEUTIC EFFECT: Prevents morbidity and death from infectious diseases

DAILY DOSAGE: 5,000–20,000 IU; the dose may be increased to 100,000 IU at the onset of flu symptoms, with another 100,000 IU taken at bedtime

VITAMIN C

THERAPEUTIC EFFECT: Improves the ability of white blood cells to fight infections and stimulates immune cells to attack viruses and cancer

DAILY DOSAGE: 2,000–6,000 mg for prevention of the common cold and pneumonia; when used to treat a cold or in conjunction with medications for pneumonia, increase the dose to just below bowel tolerance

VITAMIN E

THERAPEUTIC EFFECT: Improves certain immune system parameters, particularly augmenting antibody response and reducing upper respiratory infections

DAILY DOSAGE: 200 mg (approximately 300 IU) of natural vitamin E; higher doses (500 mg or approximately 750 IU) might yield greater therapeutic benefits

VITAMIN B_6

THERAPEUTIC EFFECT: Assists the rapidly dividing cells of the immune system and boosts production of glutathione, which is important for fighting viral infections and cancer

DAILY DOSAGE: 50–100 mg; some people might require higher doses, up to 250 mg

POLYUNSATURATED (OMEGA-3) OILS

THERAPEUTIC EFFECT: Decreases the production of inflammatory compounds and damaging free radicals

DAILY DOSAGE: 2,400 mg of EPA

ZINC

THERAPEUTIC EFFECT: Essential for all immune cells, particularly cells that are involved in fighting infections

DAILY DOSAGE: 50 mg of elemental zinc daily; the dose can be increased to 80 mg for broader therapeutic results; 1–2 mg of copper should also be taken to prevent rare blood cell abnormalities

SELENIUM

THERAPEUTIC EFFECT: Plays a critical role in guarding against oxidative damage, regulating immune function, and preventing viral and other infections

DAILY DOSAGE: 200–800 micrograms (high-selenium yeast)

PLANT STEROLS

THERAPEUTIC EFFECT: Enhances the immune response that helps to facilitate the clearance of particular pathogens, such as cold and flu viruses

DAILY DOSAGE: The sterol (BSS:BSSG) mixture should provide 20 mg of beta-sitosterol and 200 micrograms of beta-sitosterol glycoside per pill; take two pills three times daily for one month, then a maintenance dose of three pills

Summary

Immune system abnormalities are among the many dysfunctions associated with chronic fatigue. To remedy these abnormalities, people with CFS need to adopt new ways of eating, which include the elimination of dietary intolerances (food allergies), refined carbohydrates, and caffeine. They also need to eat adequate amounts of protein from healthy sources, such as wild cold-water fish and white-meat poultry without the skin. All of these dietary modifications re-balance the immune system and prevent flare-ups by reducing the incidence of infections, such as the common cold.

To support these dietary modifications, CFS sufferers should also consider supplementing with the key vitamins A, C, E, and B_6. These vitamins support the immune system, ensure that it is functioning normally, and also reduce the incidence of infections. Other important treatments should be considered, including polyunsaturated omega-3 oils, the minerals zinc and selenium, and plant sterols. These help reduce the incidence of infections and re-balance the immune system.

CHAPTER 7

TREATING MENTAL HEALTH PROBLEMS

Chronic fatigue syndrome (CFS) is strongly associated with both depression and anxiety-related symptoms.[1] The mental anguish and physical toll that anxiety and depression impose is tremendous, especially since people with CFS are already burdened by the inherent difficulties of their illness. Even though chronic fatigue is often misdiagnosed as depression, many sufferers do in fact suffer from low moods. I have also observed that there are a sizeable number of people with CFS who suffer from anxiety and feel further incapacitated by being chronically stressed, nervous, and tense.

Since it makes little sense for those with chronic fatigue to suffer needlessly from debilitating mental health symptoms, they should undergo a therapeutic trial using several of the numerous vitamin and other treatments that are available. These natural treatments usually improve quality of life and significantly reduce symptoms of chronic mental health problems.

Dietary Solutions

In Chapter 3, I recommended that people with chronic fatigue consider following an oligoantigenic (elimination) diet followed by a challenge phase to pinpoint dietary intolerances (food allergies). Once all implicated dietary items have been identified, they should be strictly avoided or ingested only once every four days to limit ongoing allergic reactions. Since food allergies can be responsible for mental health symptoms like anxiety and depression, removing ongoing allergic reactions is a vital component of an effective plan to overcome CFS.

Vitamin Solutions

Vitamin B_3

I have written extensively about the anti-anxiety effects of the form of vitamin B_3 known as niacinamide (nicotinamide).[2] It is a remarkable vitamin since it possesses many therapeutic properties that decrease symptoms of anxiety. Niacinamide is the only form of vitamin B_3 that has significant anti-anxiety properties; the other forms, NADH (nicotinamide adenine dinucleotide) and niacin (nicotinic acid), do not. Niacinamide binds near certain brain receptors, gamma-aminobutyric acid (GABA) receptors, that cause a cascade of neurochemical events to diminish symptoms of anxiety and even muscular tensions. It also reduces accumulations of lactic acid, which helps alleviate intense anxiety reactions that are usually described as "panic attacks." Reducing lactic acid also helps to ease muscle tension and pain, a common problem among many CFS sufferers. Additionally, niacinamide increases the amount of serotonin in the body and presumably in the brain. Serotonin is a "feel good" neurotransmitter that reduces symptoms of both anxiety and depression.

The majority of CFS sufferers will require a minimum of 2,000–4,500 mg of niacinamide each day to achieve therapeutic results. B_3 is so safe that daily doses in the range of 1,500–6,000 mg have been used in children and adolescents for extended periods of time without any adverse side effects or liver complications.[3] Patients should expect to feel markedly less anxiety within one month of taking this nutrient.

Because niacinamide alleviates anxiety, it can sometimes be too sedating.[4] Other potential side effects include dry mouth and nausea, but these usually disappear once the daily dose has been reduced by 500–1,000 mg. There are concerns about liver toxicity, but these are overblown, since extremely large daily doses (9,000 mg) need to be taken to cause significant liver impairment.[5] The majority of people will develop nausea and sometimes vomiting at 6,000 mg per day of niacinamide, but there is no need to go beyond 4,500 mg per day when using niacinamide to treat anxiety.[6]

Vitamin B_{12}

Vitamin B_{12} is an excellent anti-anxiety and antidepressant vitamin. Anyone with a combination of anxiety, depression, and fatigue should have their blood levels of vitamin B_{12} (serum cobalamin) measured before treatment is instituted. When initially measured, the vitamin B_{12} levels of CFS patients are typically less than 500 pmol/L. My clinical experience has shown that B_{12} levels greater than 1,000 pmol/L are necessary for people with chronic fatigue to experience relief of their anxiety, fatigue, and depression symptoms.

To get blood levels to this level quickly and safely, the optimal method is intramuscular administration of vitamin B_{12}, giving vitamin B_{12} by injection directly into the muscles of the arms, legs, or buttocks. The hydroxocobalamin form is ideal for intramuscular injection because it possesses good antioxidant effects and is retained in the body longer than the cyanocobalamin form. I teach all of my CFS patients how to administer their own vitamin B_{12} injections, which builds self-reliance and reduces their dependency on others.

Several studies demonstrate the value of providing regular vitamin B_{12} injections to patients with CFS. In one study, two subjects were randomized to receive weekly injections of hydroxocobalamin or placebo for twenty-five weeks.[7] Even though there were no statistical differences found between the hydroxocobalamin and placebo, the subjects reported a benefit from the hydroxocobalamin in terms of reduced nervousness and fatigue. In a second study, twenty-eight subjects complaining of tiredness were given injections of hydroxocobalamin (5 mg) twice weekly for two weeks, followed by a rest period of two weeks, and then a similar course of matching placebo injections. Subjects who received the placebo in the first two-week period showed a positive response to hydroxocobalamin in the second period, specifically in the categories of "general well-being" and "happiness."[8]

In another study, the effectiveness of antidepressant medications correlated with the initial levels of vitamin B_{12}. Patients who had an effective therapeutic response to their antidepressant medications had higher initial average levels of vitamin B_{12} compared to patients who did not respond and to patients that only partially responded. The authors concluded that the initial level of vitamin B_{12} in the blood "and the probability of recovery from major depression may be positively associated."[9] This finding is important since many people with chronic fatigue are taking antidepressants but are not adequately responding because their vitamin B_{12} levels are probably not optimal.

Two investigators have used vitamin B_{12} (cyanocobalamin) injections extensively on thousands of CFS patients for over ten years and have seen it benefit 50–80 percent of them.[10] Patients were given injections of 1,000 micrograms of cyanocobalamin weekly or 5,000 micrograms three times each week. Within 12–24 hours, patients noticed improvements in numbness or tingling of the extremities, abnormal gait, memory loss, weakness of the limbs, changes in mood and personality, and even fatigue. Patients needed injections of 3,000 micrograms of cyanocobalamin every 2–3 days to sustain the benefits, along with a multiple vitamin and mineral supplement containing B vitamins and folic acid (1 mg). No toxicity was seen except for the rare case of acne, which resolved when the dose was decreased.

Considering this evidence regarding the positive therapeutic value of vitamin B_{12}, chronic fatigue sufferers need to receive regular injections when trying to control their symptoms of anxiety and depression. People typically require 1,000–5,000 micrograms of intramuscular B_{12} three times a week until their mental health symptoms improve. The serum level of vitamin B_{12} should be evaluated after 4–6 weeks of treatment to make certain that it is greater than 1,000 pmol/L. The only rare side effect from intramuscular B_{12} is an acne-like eruption on the face, the upper parts of the back and chest, and even the upper arm, particularly in women. In over ten years of clinical practice, I have seen this in only a handful of patients. Once injections are discontinued, the lesions disappear within a week.

Vitamin D_3

Vitamin D_3 (cholecalciferol) has important properties that promote well-being and reduce depression. The brain uses vitamin D_3 to generate an active form of the vitamin and also contains receptors that respond to the active form.[11] A 2004 study found that a vitamin D_3 intake of 4,000 IU each day was associated with antidepressant effects.[12] The authors of this study concluded that the daily dose of 4,000 IU produced the greatest responses and its use was associated with improved well-being. A study published in 2007 evaluated vitamin D deficiency and its potential relationship to fibromyalgia. It was found that "vitamin D deficiency is common in fibromyalgia and occurs more frequently in patients with anxiety and depression."[13] Since many people with chronic fatigue suffer from fibromyalgia, and since CFS and fibromyalgia are practically indistinguishable, these findings point to an important clinical relationship between vitamin D deficiency and anxiety and depression among those with these medical syndromes.

It is probably a good idea to obtain a baseline vitamin D level (25-OH vitamin D) prior to treatment with vitamin D_3. The typical reference range is 25–100 nmol/L; however, the levels of 25-OH vitamin D should ideally be 75–125 nmol/L. This "ideal" reference range might need to be widened as research demonstrates greater health benefits with higher levels. There is an emerging body of research supporting the use of supplemental vitamin D_3 for numerous medical conditions and diseases, including mental health disorders. Even though the body produces vitamin D through exposure to sunlight, all CFS sufferers should receive supplemental vitamin D_3 regardless of their amount of time in the sun. A nontoxic and adequate daily dose of vitamin D_3 is 1,000–4,000 IU.

Folic Acid

Folic acid increases neurotransmitters, such as serotonin and dopamine, in the brain, which would account for its antidepressant effects.[14] In depressed patients unresponsive to their antidepressants, folic acid (2 mg per day) might help to improve their responses to medication.[15] This very safe dose of folic acid can be used by anyone with chronic fatigue who is on antidepressants yet continues to suffer from low moods.

Folic acid deficiency has been identified in up to one-third of all depressed inpatients.[16] For this reason, it might be a good idea for physicians to screen the blood of all their CFS patients with depression for their red cell folate status prior to treatment. A relatively common genetic defect called a polymorphism might be causally related to an increased risk of depression.[17] Individuals having this polymorphism would need to supplement with folic acid in order to prevent depression. It is conceivable that there are CFS sufferers with depression that have this polymorphism and who responded poorly to their antidepressant medications, since their folic acid requirements would be difficult to achieve from diet alone.

The recommended daily dose of folic acid is 1–5 mg. Folic acid supplementation is generally well tolerated, but in doses much higher than 2 mg each day it can be associated with increased flatulence, nausea, and loss of appetite. Supplementation should be used with extreme caution in people with chronic fatigue who also have seizure disorders.[18] Folic acid should never be supplemented without knowing vitamin B_{12} status; otherwise, there is the possibility of masking a specific anemia due to deficient levels of B_{12}. Another concern is an increased risk of prostate cancer in men that might be associated with modest folic acid supplementation.[19] Because of this, I do not recommend that my male CFS patients age 50 and older supplement with folic acid. Instead, I encourage them to eat more foods that are rich in folic acid, such as leafy green vegetables (such as spinach and lettuce), beans, peas, squash, and citrus fruits.

Other Solutions

Polyunsaturated Oils (Fats)

Polyunsaturated oils include flaxseed oil or the use of omega-3 essential fatty acids from fish. The few published studies pertaining to anxiety are promising. In one study, three out of four patients with anxiety of more than ten years' duration improved after supplementing with flaxseed oil for 2–3 months.[20] The benefits were related to an increased production of chemical compounds known as prostaglandins. Although flaxseed oil might be useful for the treatment of anxiety, it is not therapeutically equivalent to using omega-3s derived from fish[21], which are preferable because they contain eicosapentaenoic acid (EPA) and docosahexaenoic acid (DHA). These specific types of essential fatty acids have a wide spectrum of neurobehavioral effects and are more efficacious than flaxseed oil for the treatment of mental health complaints.[22]

A study found that red blood cell membrane levels of omega-3s were decreased among a group of anxiety patients.[23] This might mean that a subset of people with chronic fatigue suffering from anxiety could have deficiencies of omega-3s in their red blood cells and presumably in other tissues, such as their brains. A clinical trial assessed whether omega-3s from fish would decrease anxiety in a group of substance abusers.[24] Thirteen patients were provided with an omega-3 supplement, while another group of eleven patients was given a placebo. The patients taking the omega-3s experienced a consistent decline in their anxiety scores, which did not occur among those in the placebo group. The omega-3 fatty acids led to sustainable therapeutic effects even when they were discontinued. Supplementing with omega-3 essential fatty acids may have induced positive changes in the central nervous system.

When treating depression, it is the EPA component that is largely responsible for the well-known antidepressant effects of supplemental omega-3s from fish. EPA is known to reduce depression because it supports the neurons of the brain, improves neurotransmitter functioning, helps the neurons communicate with each other, and inhibits compounds that increase inflammation. EPA nourishes the neurons and facilitates their survival and growth throughout development.[25]

Omega-3 essential fatty acids are available in flaxseed oil and fish oils. The dose of flaxseed oil should be 2–6 tablespoons daily. Daily doses of omega-3s from fish should provide a minimum of 1 gram (1,000 mg) of EPA[26], but it is likely that higher daily doses of EPA are needed in order to produce greater therapeutic results. Supplementation with flaxseed oil can cause side effects, such as hypomania, mania, or other behavioral changes, in a very small percentage of individuals (about 3 percent).[27] Some of my patients have experienced loose stools or diarrhea from using flaxseed oil. The most common side effects from omega-3s from fish are gastrointestinal: poor digestion, belching, increased gas, diarrhea, and a fishy aftertaste. These side effects can be minimized by taking supplements with food or by using enteric-coated supplements.[28]

Glycine

Glycine is an amino acid that has therapeutic anti-anxiety properties. It works similarly to benzodiazepine medications but does not have any withdrawal or abuse associated with its use. Since receptors for glycine are found in specific regions of the brain, it has the ability to moderate symptoms of anxiety within a very short period of time. The highest concentrations of glycine are found in several brain regions, including the thalamus, amygdala, substantia nigra, putamen, and globus pallidus. When administered orally, glycine reduces the output of an adrenaline-like substance, norepinephrine, that stops anxiety and panic as well as feelings of being overwhelmed.[29]

Glycine is best taken on an empty stomach with some juice, which allows for a faster rate of absorption and quicker onset of action. People with chronic fatigue should begin with 1 teaspoon of the powder (approximately 5 grams or 5,000 mg) each day and they might need up to 40 grams (40,000 mg) to effectively reduce their anxiety. Glycine is very tasty and mixes well in juice. It can sometimes work within a few minutes, especially in situations where there is acute anxiety, such as a panic attack. Side effects, such as nausea, are very rare even when high doses are administered; most CFS sufferers will not experience any side effects.[30] Occasionally, a person with CFS might find glycine too sedating, making their fatigue much worse. In these situations, glycine might need to be stopped and other anti-anxiety treatments tried.

Gamma-Aminobutyric Acid (GABA)

Even though it works similarly to glycine, my clinical experience has shown GABA to be a more effective anti-anxiety agent for unknown reasons. I can only speculate that it probably binds more specifically to areas of the brain that reduce anxiety. There used to be uncertainty about whether GABA could cross the blood-brain barrier when administered orally, but a new natural form of GABA (PharmaGABA®) does indeed reach the brain. This new natural form has been positively shown to affect various biochemical markers of stress.[31] The recommended dose of PharmaGABA® is 100–200 mg three times a day. It is virtually free of any side effects, but there are a few reports of neurologic tingling, flushing, transient high blood pressure, and a fast heart rate in subjects taking high amounts (up to 10 grams) of a different form of GABA.[32]

5-Hydroxytryptophan (5-HTP)

Most of the therapeutic benefits of selective serotonin-reuptake inhibitor (SSRI) medications are thought to result from an increased amount of the neurotransmitter serotonin within the brain. 5-HTP is also capable of increasing the amount of serotonin in the brain, which makes this natural supplement a very good anti-anxiety and antidepressant agent, and sometimes an effective alternative to SSRIs. There are numerous clinical studies that have examined the effects of 5-HTP on depression[33], examining a total of 511 patients with different types of depression. Of these patients, 56 percent showed significant improvement while taking 5-HTP. There are also a few studies that have shown 5-HTP to help with anxiety.[34]

The optimal daily dose of 5-HTP is 200–900 mg in divided doses for at least two months.[35] The benefits might be improved by taking it with some type of carbohydrate (for example, fruit juice) on an empty stomach. Side effects are rare but can include hypomania, mild nausea, vomiting, heartburn, flatulence, feelings of fullness, and rumbling sensations.[36] Not every person with CFS responds well to 5-HTP, as there is speculation that it might worsen fatigue or gastrointestinal symptoms among some.[37] Some might want to try the amino acid L-tryptophan as an alternative to 5-HTP—it also raises serotonin levels and should have a similar efficacy. However, I am not convinced of this and have found L-tryptophan to be inferior to 5-HTP, which is a more direct precursor to serotonin and appears to work better.

Rhodiola Rosea

The herb *Rhodiola rosea* is commonly used in traditional medical systems in eastern Europe and Asia. It possesses both antidepressant and anti-anxiety properties and can even be used alongside any mainstream psychotropic medication. I have been impressed with its clinical utility among many of my anxious CFS patients. It seems to work fairly fast and is virtually free of side effects, even among the most sensitive patients. Rarely, a person might experience an increase in irritability and insomnia within several days of use.[38] In a clinical study involving anxious patients, *Rhodiola* extract (340 mg) for ten weeks resulted in significant declines in anxiety, as assessed by the Hamilton Anxiety Rating Scale.[39] These results were comparable to those from mainstream drugs in similar clinical trials evaluating anxiety. Other studies have found *Rhodiola* extract to significantly reduce symptoms of depression.[40]

The herb's mechanism is not well understood. It does influence the levels of serotonin, dopamine, and norepinephrine in the brain, and it also restores sensitivity to cortisol within the body.[41] This latter mechanism is important because abnormal function of the hypothalamic-pituitary-adrenal axis, and therefore dysregulated cortisol, is linked to chronic fatigue.[42]

The typical daily dose range is 340–680 mg of *Rhodiola* extract (standardized to 3 percent rosavins, the herb's active constituent). When using the herb chronically, one source recommends week-long intervals of abstinence[43], but I have not observed any dangers or reduction in therapeutic response when it is taken continually.

St. John's Wort Extract

St. John's wort is an herb that increases the amount of serotonin within the brain. Many people with CFS are given SSRI medications because increasing the levels of serotonin in the brain helps with their symptoms of anxiety and depression. St. John's wort works similarly to mainstream antidepressant SSRIs with fewer side effects.[44] It has also shown to be efficacious for the treatment of anxiety.[45] In two randomized clinical trials, it even alleviated symptoms of somatoform disorder, a psychiatric condition marked by anxiety and worry over the perception that there is something physically wrong.[46] Based on the available evidence, there appears to be a reasonable body of literature demonstrating therapeutic equivalency between St. John's wort extract and SSRIs. Even so, there are clinical concerns with its use: St. John's wort influences a specific enzyme in the liver that metabolizes most medications, which explains why there are so many potential drug interactions when it is taken in conjunction with other drugs.[47]

An effective daily dose of St. John's wort extract is 600–2,400 mg. Any CFS sufferer who takes St. John's wort must be closely monitored for drug interactions and possible, albeit rare, side effects of dry mouth, sensitivity to the sun, and gastrointestinal disturbances.

Ginkgo Biloba Extract (GBE)

Ginkgo extract appears to influence several neurotransmitters involved in mood, such as noradrenaline and serotonin. A clinical trial using several different doses of ginkgo found them to be highly effective for the treatment of anxiety: the high-dose extract (480 mg each day) was superior to the low-dose extract (240 mg each day), and both dosages produced more significant anti-anxiety effects than placebo.[48] Ginkgo also possesses antidepressant effects. A clinical study found GBE to be helpful among depressed patients with sleep disturbances.[49] The extract specifically helped to ameliorate the deficient non-REM component of sleep. This is important since sleep disturbances and depression are common problems among people with chronic fatigue.

The daily dose of *Ginkgo biloba* extract to try is in the range of 240–480 mg. GBE should be standardized to 24 percent flavone glycosides and 6 percent terpene lactones. Side effects are rare, but some of my patients have reported rashes, nausea, and dizziness that cease once it is discontinued. For CFS sufferers on blood-thinning medications, the use of ginkgo must be closely monitored by an experienced clinician.

Valerian Extract

The herb valerian has been traditionally used to help with insomnia, but it has a better spectrum of clinical efficacy when used to alleviate anxiety. I have found it to work as well as benzodiazepines, which are commonly prescribed anti-anxiety medications. Benzodiazepines are extremely difficult to withdraw from, but valerian does not create the same type of physical dependency. Valerian works by increasing the neurotransmitter GABA, which is responsible for its anti-anxiety properties.[50] Animal experiments have found valerian to not only possess anti-anxiety properties but to have antidepressant properties as well.[51]

For the treatment of anxiety, I typically recommend 800–1,600 mg of valerian (an extract standardized to 0.8 percent valeric acid). The side effect of increased or worsened fatigue is possible when it is given to people with chronic fatigue, which would necessitate a lowering of the daily dose. It can sometimes cause gastrointestinal disturbances, but these types of symptoms are fairly rare.

Probiotics

Probiotics are friendly bacteria that improve the health of the small and large intestines, reduce allergies, and alleviate symptoms of irritable bowel syndrome. A recent study has determined that probiotics can reduce symptoms of anxiety.[52] Thirty-nine patients with chronic fatigue were given daily supplementation with either a probiotic (providing 24 billion colony-forming units of *Lactobacillus casei*) or placebo for two months. At the conclusion of the study, those who took the probiotic supplement had significant reductions in their symptoms of anxiety. It is not known just how probiotics influence anxiety, but they might be capable of altering brain chemicals, such as serotonin and dopamine.[53] Probiotics might also influence how emotions (such as anxiety) are processed by directly communicating with specific areas of the brain through gut-brain interactions. Since the probiotic treatment was without any side effects, this intervention should be considered for all people with CFS.

An effective dose of probiotics is capsules that provide 24 billion colony-forming units daily. Although the study did not mention side effects, it is possible that some people might experience some gas and bloating during the first several days of treatment.

Case History

A forty-six-year-old woman presented to the Robert Schad Naturopathic Clinic (Toronto, Ontario) in October 2007. She described a long-standing history of chronic fatigue, which began twelve years previously. Besides significant fatigue, she also suffered from severe depression (major depressive disorder) and anxiety. She was taking two prescription medications, Remeron® (mirtazapine) for depression and Klonopin (clonazepam) for anxiety. Her goal was to wean off the clonazepam and maintain the other medication since she felt the antidepressant was necessary. This patient believed that the majority of her CFS symptoms were worsened by clonazepam, which is a common anti-anxiety drug (benzodiazepine). Even with our help, she was unable to get off the medication, which contributed significantly to her ongoing problems. After about six weeks, she became extremely frustrated and stopped coming to the clinic.

I included this case to highlight a common problem that I see when people with CFS are placed on clonazepam or similar anti-anxiety medications. The major concern with benzodiazepines is that dependence can develop from chronic use, as had occurred in this case. *Dependence* refers to the withdrawal symptoms from discontinuing the anti-anxiety medication, including anxiety, irritability, and insomnia, which make it extremely difficult for patients to ever get off them. Additional problems from benzodiazepines include discontinuation side effects, such as impairments in verbal memory, motor control/performance, and nonverbal memory, which can occur long after they are stopped.

This is devastating because these medications not only cause significant withdrawal symptoms but contribute to ongoing cognitive disturbances, which are unfortunately a common manifestation of chronic fatigue. Chronic use of benzodiazepines can also dampen feelings and emotions. Because clonazepam and other benzodiazepines can significantly worsen the chances of recovering from CFS, I urge all patients and their clinicians to try the vitamin and other options described in this chapter prior to using a benzodiazepine. None of these natural treatments blunt emotions nor do they produce similar types of withdrawal symptoms and discontinuation side effects.

TREATING MENTAL HEALTH PROBLEMS

OLIGOANTIGENIC (ELIMINATION) DIET

THERAPEUTIC EFFECT: To identify and reduce dietary intolerances (food allergies)

DAILY DOSAGE: Follow a diet that does not contain any implicated dietary items (food allergens), or a rotation diet in which the foods are ingested infrequently

NIACINAMIDE

THERAPEUTIC EFFECT: Alleviates anxiety by stimulating GABA receptors, reducing accumulations of lactic acid, and increasing the production of serotonin

DAILY DOSAGE: 2,000–4,500 mg niacinamide

VITAMIN B_{12}

THERAPEUTIC EFFECT: Alleviates anxiety and depression by increasing the B_{12} level in the blood and likely the brain

DAILY DOSAGE: 1,000–5,000 micrograms three times per week given intramuscularly (hydroxocobalamin preferred; cyanocobalamin fine to use, but not as effective)

VITAMIN D_3

THERAPEUTIC EFFECT: Alleviates depression and possibly anxiety by correcting vitamin D deficiency in the blood

DAILY DOSAGE: 1,000–4,000 IU cholecalciferol

FOLIC ACID

THERAPEUTIC EFFECT: Alleviates depression by increasing the production of neurotransmitters by correcting for deficiency

DAILY DOSAGE: 1–5 mg; vitamin B_{12} blood levels need to be evaluated prior to supplementation

POLYUNSATURATED OILS

THERAPEUTIC EFFECT: Alleviate both depression and anxiety by increasing omega-3 essential fatty acids in the blood

DAILY DOSAGE: 2–6 tablespoons of flaxseed oil; 1,000 mg of EPA from fish

GLYCINE

THERAPEUTIC EFFECT: Reduces anxiety through therapeutic effects similar to benzodiazepine drugs

DAILY DOSAGE: 5–40 grams mixed in juice and taken between meals

GABA

THERAPEUTIC EFFECT: Reduces anxiety through therapeutic effects similar to benzodiazepine drugs

DAILY DOSAGE: 300–600 mg

5-HTP

THERAPEUTIC EFFECT: Reduces anxiety and depression by increasing the amount of serotonin in the brain

DAILY DOSAGE: 200–900 mg

RHODIOLA ROSEA

THERAPEUTIC EFFECT: Reduces anxiety and depression by influencing neurotransmitters and increasing sensitivity to cortisol

DAILY DOSAGE: 340–680 mg

ST. JOHN'S WORT EXTRACT

THERAPEUTIC EFFECT: Reduces anxiety and depression by increasing the amount of serotonin in the brain

DAILY DOSAGE: 600–2,400 mg

GINKGO BILOBA EXTRACT

THERAPEUTIC EFFECT: Reduces anxiety and depression by influencing several neurotransmitters involved in mood

DAILY DOSAGE: 240–480 mg

VALERIAN EXTRACT

THERAPEUTIC EFFECT: Reduces anxiety through therapeutic effects similar to benzodiazepine drugs

DAILY DOSAGE: 800–1,600 mg

PROBIOTICS

THERAPEUTIC EFFECT: Reduces anxiety by possibly altering brain levels of dopamine and serotonin and by influencing areas of the brain involved in emotions

DAILY DOSAGE: 24 billion colony-forming units of *Lactobacilli* species

Summary

The extra burden that chronic fatigue sufferers experience with the added stress of anxiety and depression only makes their daily life more challenging and overwhelming. The therapeutic use of vitamin and other treatments provides hope to those with CFS searching for ways to help themselves psychologically. Effective vitamin treatments with anti-anxiety properties include vitamins B_3 and B_{12}. Vitamin therapies for depression include folic acid and vitamin D_3. Other natural compounds that possess anti-anxiety or antidepressant properties include GABA, glycine, 5-HTP, *Rhodiola rosea,* St. John's wort, *Ginkgo biloba,* valerian, and probiotics. All of these vitamin and other treatments have helped many people with CFS overcome their debilitating symptoms and live a more "normal" life. While these treatments do not necessarily cure people of their mental health struggles, they allow them to live a happier and healthier life.

CHAPTER 8

ALLEVIATING MUSCULAR DYSFUNCTION

People with chronic fatigue syndrome (CFS) typically complain of muscle aches and pains (referred to as myalgias in the medical literature), as well as muscular fatigue and weakness. Since muscular dysfunction is such a common problem among many with CFS, natural treatments should be instituted to not only reduce muscle pain but to also increase the ability to perform daily activities, such as walking, completing household chores, and simply moving around. Carrying out these common activities depends on a normal and healthy muscular system.

Research confirms the likely relationship between chronic fatigue and muscular dysfunction. One CFS case documented early intracellular acidosis (a state in which there is not enough oxygen) following moderate exercise.[1] Another, decades-old study evaluated clinical, pathological, electrophysiological, immunological, and virological abnormalities in fifty patients with postviral fatigue syndrome.[2] Many of the patients demonstrated prolonged weakness in several bodily areas (arms and legs) following specific exercises. Muscle biopsies were performed on twenty of the patients and the results demonstrated necrosis (death) in many muscle fibers, as well as evidence of early intracellular acidosis. A more recent study found an increased amount of oxidative stress and marked alterations of muscle function among chronic fatigue patients who were subjected to incremental exercise.[3]

All of these studies demonstrate the presence of muscular dysfunction, and thus explain the observed clinical findings among CFS sufferers, such as muscle weakness, post-exercise fatigue, and muscle pain.

Dietary Solutions

In Chapter 3, I recommended that people with chronic fatigue consider following an oligoantigenic (elimination) diet, followed by a challenge phase to pinpoint dietary intolerances (food allergies). Once all implicated dietary items have been identified, they should be strictly avoided or ingested only once every four days to limit ongoing allergic reactions. Since dietary items can be responsible for troubling muscular symptoms like joint pain and chronic muscle tension, removing ongoing allergic reactions is a vital component of an effective plan to overcome CFS.

Vitamin Solutions

Vitamin D_3

There is speculation that the muscle pain of chronic fatigue and fibromyalgia might be related to a deficiency in vitamin D[4], which has also been implicated in muscle weakness and fatigue. It is probably wise to obtain a baseline vitamin D (25-OH vitamin D) level prior to treatment with vitamin D_3 (cholecalciferol). The typical reference range is 25–100 nmol/L; however, the levels of 25-OH vitamin D should ideally be 75–125 nmol/L for optimal results. This "ideal" reference range might need to be widened as more research demonstrates greater health benefits with higher vitamin D levels.

Vitamin D is produced in the body with exposure to sunlight. However, all CFS sufferers should take supplemental vitamin D_3 regardless of their exposures to the sun. A safe, non-toxic, and adequate daily dose of D_3 is 1,000–4,000 IU.

Other Solutions

Acetyl-L-Carnitine (ALC)

ALC is a naturally occurring substance capable of crossing the blood-brain barrier and increasing brain levels of acetylcholine, a chemical involved in learning and memory. ALC also increases blood flow, enhances the activity of certain enzymes, and increases energy metabolism in the brain.[5]

A study published in 2007 evaluated the therapeutic effects of ALC among patients having fibromyalgia syndrome, a condition very similar to chronic fatigue.[6] In fact, I believe both CFS and fibromyalgia syndrome to be the same clinical entity, with the only difference between the syndromes (although this is the subject of much debate) being that fibromyalgia is characterized by more profound muscle pain. The reason for using ALC was the assumption that fibromyalgia patients might be deficient in carnitine, which is influenced by ALC. Patients were given two capsules (totaling 1,000 mg) each day of either ALC or placebo, and they were also given one intramuscular injection of either ALC (500 mg) or placebo. The dosages were increased after two weeks to three capsules (totaling 1,500 mg) daily for eight weeks. The fibromyalgia patients who took the ALC had improvements in depression and musculoskeletal pain. The ALC was well tolerated and no serious side effects were reported.

These findings are important considering a previous study demonstrated that ALC (2,000 mg) alleviated both general and mental fatigue among a group of CFS patients.[7] The changes in blood levels of carnitine correlated with the clinical improvements. Specifically, blood levels of carnitine were inversely related to symptom relief—the least increase was associated with the greatest improvement. It was hypothesized that those who responded to ALC had a better ability to transport carnitine from the blood into their tissues, such as the brain.

The study results support ALC as an intervention to reduce the muscular dysfunction and fatigue associated with chronic fatigue.

The optimal therapeutic dose is 2,000 mg daily. There is no need to worry about side effects since ALC is virtually free of them.

Magnesium and Malic Acid

There is some degree of tissue hypoxia (oxygen deprivation) among both fibromyalgia and chronic fatigue patients, and this hypoxia is related to abnormal levels of the mineral magnesium and possibly malic acid (an organic compound found in many tart or sour foods). Since all tissues of the body depend on adequate oxygen, it is not surprising that magnesium and malic acid help. Both nutrients support energy production within the cells, which might naturally reverse some biochemical manifestations of oxygen deprivation, such as muscular fatigue and pain.

Disordered metabolism of the mineral magnesium appears to play a role in the pathogenesis of both chronic fatigue and fibromyalgia. Data shows that people with CFS had higher magnesium levels compared to normal individuals.[8] The significance of this finding is not known, but I suspect it has something to do with poor muscular utilization of magnesium. A previous study identified deficiencies of magnesium within the cells of chronic fatigue patients despite normal blood levels.[9] Abnormal intracellular concentrations of calcium and magnesium were found in fibromyalgia patients but not in healthy individuals.[10] This abnormality may be responsible for the symptom of muscular tension, which is so common among people with fibromyalgia.

One clinical study used 300–600 mg of magnesium and 1,200–2,400 mg of malic acid in fifteen patients with fibromyalgia for an average of eight weeks.[11] All patients experienced subjective improvements and decreased tender points (specific areas of muscular pain). Another study found that the highest daily doses of magnesium (300 mg) and malic acid (1,200 mg) were more effective in reducing symptoms of muscle pain and tenderness when compared to lower daily doses.[12]

The effective initial daily dose of magnesium is 300 mg and the dose for malic acid is 1,200 mg. After two months, if there are no clear benefits, you may want to try doubling each dose. Good supplemental and highly absorbable forms of magnesium include magnesium citrate and magnesium glycinate. Other less effective and poorly absorbable forms of supplemental magnesium include magnesium gluconate and magnesium oxide. When looking at the labels of magnesium supplements, be certain to check the amount of elemental magnesium that is delivered per pill. The elemental dose refers to the amount of magnesium that can be effectively absorbed. For example, if the label shows 600 mg of magnesium glycinate, the elemental amount will usually also be listed as 120 mg. A label may also simply state the amount of magnesium per pill: "Magnesium (as magnesium citrate) 160 mg." The dose of magnesium specified here refers to the elemental amounts.

There are usually no side effects from magnesium, but loose stools and diarrhea might result when using daily doses above 300 mg. If these side effects develop, the dose should be lowered by 50–100 mg. While there is a lack of clinical information pertaining to side effects from malic acid, it does appear to be relatively free from any untoward effects. The only side effect reported in one study was diarrhea when higher malic acid dosages were used. This was, however, most likely due to the magnesium component of the magnesium-malic acid formula under evaluation.

5-Hydroxytryptophan (5-HTP)

As a precursor to the neurotransmitter serotonin, 5-HTP might be capable of reducing the sensation of muscular pain. One of the potential causes of fibromyalgia (and perhaps chronic fatigue) is decreased flux through the serotonin pathway.[13] Two clinical studies demonstrated that 5-HTP improved symptoms of anxiety, pain intensity, quality of sleep, fatigue, and number of tender points among fibromyalgia patients.[14] As both CFS and fibromyalgia are closely related, it is possible that 5-HTP would yield similar results in people with chronic fatigue.

A report discussing both CFS and fibromyalgia made specific reference to disturbances in brain chemistry and the therapeutic effectiveness of mainstream psychotropic medications that specifically increase serotonin.[15] Serotonin-increasing agents decrease the sensation of pain, and 5-HTP has a similar mechanism of action. Thus, it makes sense to try 5-HTP in chronic fatigue to see if it alleviates muscular pain.

The optimal daily dose of 5-HTP is 300 mg in divided doses. Absorption might be improved by taking 5-HTP with some type of carbohydrate (such as fruit juice) on an empty stomach. Side effects of 5-HTP are rare, but can include hypomania, mild nausea, vomiting, heartburn, flatulence, feelings of fullness, and rumbling sensations.[16] Not every person with CFS responds well to 5-HTP, as it might worsen fatigue or gastrointestinal symptoms in some.[17]

D-Ribose

D-ribose is a natural substance that increases cellular energy within muscle tissue, making it a suitable intervention for the muscular dysfunctions associated with chronic fatigue. In a clinical study, forty-one patients with fibromyalgia and/or CFS were given D-ribose (5 grams) three times daily.[18] Each patient ingested a total of 280 grams of D-ribose during the clinical trial. Overall, D-ribose was well tolerated and patients showed improvements in their sleep, mental clarity, pain intensity, and well-being. Specifically, there was a 66 percent improvement overall, a 45 percent improvement in energy, and an overall improvement in well-being of 30 percent.

The typical therapeutic dose of D-ribose is 5 grams three times daily, taken with juice or a meal. There are seldom any side effects from D-ribose supplementation. Should they develop, they are typically gastrointestinal in nature and will abate when the daily dose is decreased by 5 grams.

ALLEVIATING MUSCULAR DYSFUNCTION

OLIGOANTIGENIC (ELIMINATION) DIET

THERAPEUTIC EFFECT: To identify and reduce dietary intolerances (food allergies)

DAILY DOSAGE: Follow a diet that does not contain any implicated dietary items or a rotation diet in which the dietary items are ingested infrequently

VITAMIN D_3

THERAPEUTIC EFFECT: Alleviates muscular weakness and pain, particularly when there is laboratory evidence of deficiency

DAILY DOSAGE: 1,000–4,000 IU cholecalciferol

ACETYL-L-CARNITINE (ALC)

THERAPEUTIC EFFECT: Modifies the utilization of carnitine, which decreases muscular pain

DAILY DOSAGE: 2,000 mg

MAGNESIUM AND MALIC ACID

THERAPEUTIC EFFECT: Supports energy production within cells and reverses symptoms of oxygen deprivation, including muscular fatigue and pain

DAILY DOSAGE: 300–600 mg of elemental magnesium and 1,200–2,400 mg of malic acid

5-HYDROXYTRYPTOPHAN (5-HTP)

THERAPEUTIC EFFECT: Reduces muscular pain by increasing the amount of serotonin in the brain

DAILY DOSAGE: 300 mg

D-RIBOSE

THERAPEUTIC EFFECT: Increases cellular energy within muscle tissue

DAILY DOSAGE: 5 grams three times daily (take with juice or a meal)

Summary

Muscular dysfunction is a common problem among people with chronic fatigue, who often suffer from muscular fatigue and pain, possibly due to several factors, including vitamin D deficiency, impaired carnitine utilization, abnormal magnesium levels, and serotonin abnormalities. The use of specific vitamin (vitamin D_3) and other treatments (acetyl-L-carnitine, magnesium and malic acid, 5-hydroxytryptophan, and D-ribose) help to alleviate these debilitating symptoms and restore a reasonable quality of life for those with chronic fatigue.

CHAPTER 9

TREATING RED BLOOD CELL ABNORMALITIES AND OXIDATIVE STRESS

The relationship between impaired microcirculatory blood flow and chronic fatigue syndrome (CFS) is a neglected area of inquiry. Normal tissue function depends on an adequate supply of oxygen and metabolic substrates, which is only possible in the presence of normal capillary blood flow. Capillaries are tiny blood vessels that carry oxygenated blood to the tissues of the body. Since many of the smaller capillaries in the human body have diameters that are more narrow than the diameters of red blood cells (RBCs), adequate perfusion of bodily tissues depends on the ability of RBCs to change from their normal discocyte shape (a process called deformation) so that they can readily traverse (enter into) the capillaries.[1]

Numerous studies have evaluated microcirculatory blood flow and/or RBC deformability in subjects with chronic fatigue. In a study comparing blood filterability, samples of blood from acutely unwell CFS subjects were shown to be less filterable than blood from similarly aged blood donors.[2] These subjects had prolonged blood filtration times that normalized to that of the aged blood donors once their acute illnesses had passed. Based on these findings, the investigators concluded that the numerous symptoms of chronic fatigue might result from impaired microcirculatory blood flow. A 1987 report discovered abnormal RBC shape changes among chronic fatigue patients in a state of relapse.[3] The cell membranes of the altered RBCs were thought to be more rigid, thus impairing the delivery of oxygen and other nutrient materials.

In another study, blood samples from 102 CFS patients, 99 multiple sclerosis patients, and 52 healthy controls were compared.[4] Chronic fatigue patients had the highest percentage of non-discocytic (abnormally shaped) RBCs and the lowest percentage of normal RBCs. There was an inverse correlation between the number of non-discocytic RBCs and well-being among the chronic fatigue patients. It was concluded that these results show evidence of an organic cause of chronic fatigue. In a similar study, individuals suffering from chronic tiredness and easy fatigability also had increased numbers (higher percentages) of non-discocytic red blood cells.[5]

One study evaluated RBC shapes from 620 male and 1,558 female members of CFS organizations from New Zealand, Australia, South Africa, and England.[6] When compared to a group of healthy individuals from New Zealand, the results showed a much higher percentage of flat cells among the members of the CFS organizations. Since flat cells do not deform well, this would adversely affect blood function and consequently capillary blood flow. A similar study with blood samples from 632 American subjects (most of whom had chronic fatigue or some variant of it) demonstrated a greater percentage of flat cells among all the subjects.[7]

The implications of these studies are tremendous since they point to a common abnormal finding—abnormal RBC shape changes—among individuals with chronic fatigue and related disorders. The clinical consequences of having abnormally shaped red blood cells include the following:

- Impaired deformability of RBCs
- Reduced rate of capillary (microcirculatory) blood flow
- Reduced capacity to load and release oxygen
- The presence of small areas of ischemic necrosis (damage due to an absence of oxygen) within the small capillaries of the body[8]

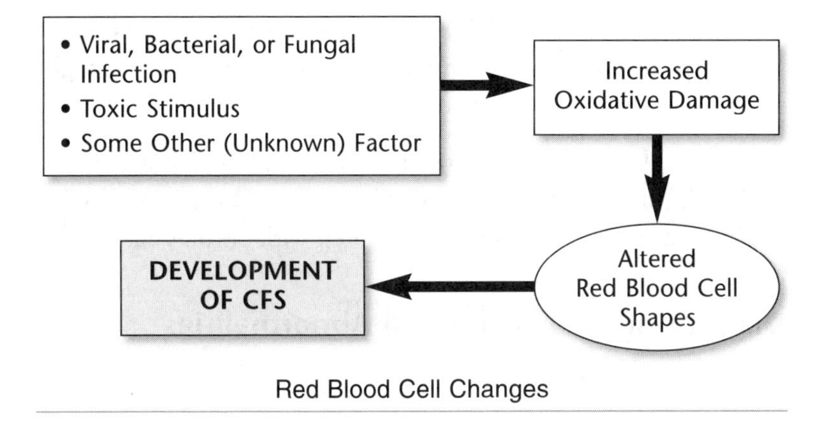

Red Blood Cell Changes

This would account for the unrelenting tiredness, post-exertional malaise, and central nervous system dysfunction that all CFS patients experience. An insufficient supply of oxygen and nutrient substrates would eventually lead to recognizable clinical findings apparent to any examining clinician.

Triggering events such as viral infections, bacterial infections, or exposure to a toxic stimulus could have perturbed the RBC environment leading to shape transformations.[9] More recent data, however, has identified oxidative stress as the likely cause of altered red blood cell shapes among those with chronic fatigue.[10] In one study, blood samples from thirty-one CFS patients were compared to forty-one healthy control subjects. The red blood cells from all the samples were examined and classified according to their shapes. In addition, blood measurements of specific markers of oxidative stress were taken, including RBC malondialdehyde (MDA), RBC glutathione (GSH), 2,3-diphosphoglycerate (2,3-DPG), and methemoglobin (MetHb). The results demonstrated statistically significant differences in several parameters, with the chronic fatigue group having significantly increased levels of RBC MDA, 2,3-DPG, and MetHb compared to the control group. These results explain some of the reasons why altered RBC shapes create problems for people with chronic fatigue:

- Elevated levels of 2,3-DPG increase RBC fragility and decrease deformability

- Elevated levels of MetHb are indicative of increased oxidative damage to the hemoglobin molecule, which leads to damaged RBC membranes and reduced deformability
- Elevated levels of MDA are indicative of oxidative damage to the RBC membranes, which contributes to the decreased deformability and altered function associated with chronic fatigue.[11]

Diagnosing Red Blood Cell Abnormalities

At present, there are no laboratories, outside of one academic institution, that have been evaluating red blood cell shape changes in chronic fatigue. Some patients and clinicians might believe that "live blood cell analysis" would yield similar information and be capable of demonstrating abnormally shaped RBCs. To my knowledge, there are no studies that have relied on live blood cell analysis to determine RBC shape abnormalities. All of the studies cited above used a specialized technique of collecting and processing blood samples. As far as I know, there is no current laboratory that collects blood samples and sends reports. Until such a service becomes available, it seems prudent to simply assume that abnormally shaped RBCs accompany chronic fatigue.

Dietary Solutions

In Chapter 3, I recommended that people with chronic fatigue consider following an oligoantigenic (elimination) diet, followed by a challenge phase to pinpoint dietary intolerances (food allergies). Once all implicated dietary items have been identified, they should be strictly avoided or ingested only once every four days to limit ongoing allergic reactions. Since dietary items can be responsible for increasing free radical production and oxidative damage (for example, from ingesting fried and/or processed foods), removing food allergens is a vital component of an effective plan to overcome CFS.

Vitamin Solutions

Vitamin B_{12} (Hydroxocobalamin)

The fact that oxidative stress leads to altered RBC shape changes helps us in identifying therapeutically valuable treatments. Vitamin B_{12} functions as an antioxidant, since it scavenges nitric oxide and helps to normalize excessive amounts of both nitric oxide and peroxynitrite free radicals.[12] It probably exerts its beneficial effects by stopping oxidative damage to the blood cell membranes. Injectable B_{12} has been shown to normalize RBC shapes in approximately 50 percent of chronic fatigue patients given the vitamin.[13] Twenty-eight patients with "acute" or new-onset CFS were each administered 1 mg (1,000 micrograms) of injectable hydroxocobalamin. The patients who symtomatically improved were found to have reduced numbers of abnormally shaped RBCs and responded within twenty-four hours.

When using injectable vitamin B_{12} for chronic fatigue, there should be an improvement within twenty-four hours of receiving the treatment. The symptoms will inevitably return, and when they do another injection is needed. There are instances in which CFS sufferers have lived virtually normal lifestyles while receiving B_{12} injections at 12–20 day intervals.[14] The reason for the effectiveness of B_{12} in only 50 percent of cases is unknown.

I have used injectable vitamin B_{12} in numerous cases and have generally found it to help patients live a better quality of life with more energy, less post-exertional malaise, fewer cognitive disturbances, and improved mental health. Since the frequency of injections depends on each person's response, I have found that some require one injection each month while others need 3–5 injections each week. I teach each CFS patient how to self-inject so that treatment can be individualized for optimal outcomes.

The dose of vitamin B_{12} might need to be increased from 1 mg to 3–5 mg (3,000–5,000 micrograms) per injection several times each week. There is published data demonstrating excellent results when using very high doses of injectable B_{12}.[15] There should not be any concern about side effects or about the high blood levels of B_{12} from frequent injections. In over ten years of clinical practice, I have only seen a handful of patients experience a self-limiting acne-like eruption from vitamin B_{12} injections.

Vitamin C

Vitamin C is a water-soluble antioxidant with potent healing properties. It has been shown to reverse red blood cell shape changes and increase RBC function when administered at doses of 15 grams intravenously to chronically disabled CFS patients.[16] Although giving vitamin C orally will not raise blood levels to the degree that intravenous vitamin C does, optimal therapeutic doses of oral vitamin C might be capable of also normalizing the RBC shapes and function. An effective oral dose of vitamin C ranges from 1,000 to 12,000 mg daily. If diarrhea occurs, simply reducing the dose by 500–1,000 mg should resolve the issue.

Vitamin E

Vitamin E possesses considerable antioxidant activity and protects blood cell membranes from oxidative damage.[17] Recommended therapeutic doses of vitamin E are in the range of 400 to 1,200 IU each day of natural D-alpha tocopherol.

Other Solutions

Polyunsaturated Oils (Fats)

Polyunsaturated oils include both evening primrose oil and fish oil. Evening primrose oil is a potentially valuable treatment for people with chronic fatigue that contains gamma-linolenic acid (GLA), an essential nutrient having important therapeutic properties. GLA is an omega-6 essential fatty acid, so it must be obtained from dietary sources or converted within the body from dietary sources of linoleic acid. The conversion of linoleic acid to GLA requires the delta-6-desaturase enzyme, which can become impaired as a result of aging, diabetes, viral infections, and even radiotherapy.[18] A report in 2007 linked some of the signs and symptoms of CFS to delta-6-desaturase enzymatic damage, possibly resulting from a persistent viral infection.[19] Being able to generate enough GLA in the body is necessary for the synthesis of prostaglandin E1 (PGE1), which in turn increases the functioning of the red blood cells. Evening primrose oil as a source of GLA appears to be effective in 70 percent of CFS cases.[20] The typical therapeutic dose of evening primrose oil is 4,000 mg per day, based on a study that demonstrated significant increases in PGE1 among patients with eczema.[21]

If no observable benefits occur after six weeks of using evening primrose oil, it should be stopped and replaced with fats derived from fish oil. Fish oils contain the omega-3 essential fatty acids eicosapentaenoic acid (EPA) and docosahexaenoic acid (DHA). It is likely the EPA component that produces favorable effects on blood cell membranes. Although the body converts dietary sources of omega-3s into EPA, the conversion is thought to be impaired among CFS sufferers since it requires the normal function of delta-6-desaturase enzymes. An insufficient amount of dietary omega-3s might even cause chronic fatigue and lead to immunological defects.[22] Since fish oil sources increase the production of prostaglandins of the 3-series, they positively influence blood cell membrane functions[23] and have been shown to reduce the percentage of abnormally shaped RBCs when given orally.[24]

Thus, it makes logical sense to try fish oil supplementation when previous treatment with evening primrose oil is not successful. I recommend liquid sources of fish oil that contain a higher ratio of EPA to DHA. I generally start with 1,500 mg of EPA and 500 mg of DHA and observe my patients over the course of 6–8 weeks. If there is no apparent therapeutic result, additional nutritional treatments should be tried.

Glutathione

Depletion of the antioxidant glutathione is associated with increased blood-brain permeability, causing unwanted molecules and other substances to enter the brain.[25] Taking supplemental glutathione would directly increase its levels in the blood and possibly within the red blood cells as well. A study using a special (liposomal) form of glutathione demonstrated powerful antioxidant effects against oxidative damage.[26] A liposomal glutathione preparation (ReadiSorb™ Liposomal Glutathione) appears to be capable of raising RBC glutathione levels. Typical therapeutic doses are 1.0–1.5 teaspoons per day, providing approximately 420–600 mg of glutathione.

Alpha-Lipoic Acid (ALA)

Alpha-lipoic acid is a unique antioxidant that has the capability of indirectly raising glutathione levels.[27] It also helps to regenerate both vitamins C and E. Supplemental doses of alpha-lipoic acid should be in the range of 150–300 mg daily.

Ginkgo Biloba Extract

The use of *Ginkgo biloba* extract should be considered because of its specific compounds flavonoids and terpenoids, which have biological properties that positively influence the functioning of red blood cells. The typical daily dose of ginkgo is 60–240 mg of an extract standardized to 24 percent flavone glycosides and 6 percent terpene lactones. Side effects with ginkgo are rare, but some of my patients have reported rashes, nausea, and dizziness that cease once it is discontinued.

Vinpocetine

Vinpocetine possesses significant free radical scavenging ability, which would possibly limit oxidative damage to the blood cell membranes. It also has therapeutic properties that improve capillary blood flow and the delivery of oxygen and nutrients to the organs and tissues.[28] The typical dose of vinpocetine is 10 mg three times daily. Its side effect profile is comparable to ginkgo.

Gamma-Aminobutyric Acid, Glycine, Vitamin B_3, and 5-Hydroxytryptophan

These treatments—gamma-aminobutyric acid (GABA), glycine, vitamin B_3, and 5-hydroxytryptophan (5-HTP)—have been addressed previously (see Chapter 7), but they can be used therapeutically to resolve abnormal RBC shape changes among chronic fatigue sufferers. Their benefits are directly related to their anti-stress and anti-anxiety properties. When individuals are stressed or anxious, they secrete chemicals called catecholamines, which have been shown to decrease RBC function and increase the stickiness or thickness of blood.[29] Thus, any of these nutrients would be helpful because they would be capable of limiting the release of catecholamines. Both GABA and glycine possess effects that might mimic those of benzodiazepine (anti-anxiety) medications. B_3 (niacinamide) also influences the benzodiazepine system within the brain and would be able to limit the stress response. 5-HTP is a precursor to serotonin and would therefore increase the amount of this beneficial neurotransmitter within the brain. The only caution when using 5-HTP is that some data indicates a potential to worsen fatigue or gastrointestinal symptoms among those with CFS.[30] The recommended dosages and possible side effects of these nutrients can be found in Chapter 7.

Case Histories

A fifty-six-year-old woman visited me for an evaluation in May 2002 after she was given a diagnosis of chronic fatigue syndrome by a previous clinician.[31] Her history revealed debilitating tiredness, which she rated a 7–8/10, with 10 being the worst. Her sleep was inadequate, only 4–7 hours each night, and she never felt refreshed in the morning. Her tiredness was worsened by walking up and down stairs and doing mild activities of daily living. Naps seemed to help, but they interfered with her quality of life because she needed several of them each day. She also complained of muscle weakness and forgetfulness that had recently become obvious to other people. She was on disability from work due to her current state of health. Her physical examination was normal, and there were no neurological or muscular deficits. She noted that vitamin B_{12} injections had helped her in the past, and she was given another injection of B_{12} and was taught how to self-administer injections. When she returned for a follow-up visit in June, she was happy with her progress and was now able to walk up or down two flights of stairs without difficulty. Her brain no longer felt "fogged-up" and she was able to resume work. People even commented that her memory seemed better. Against my advice, she discontinued the B_{12} injections. In July, the patient called and reported that her symptoms had worsened, especially the tiredness, and I obviously recommended that she resume the B_{12} injections. When she returned in August, she reported having significant improvements from resuming the vitamin B_{12} injections. Her tiredness had improved, rating a 1–2/10, and the fogginess and memory problems were also gone.

In a second case, a forty-five-year-old woman began receiving injections of vitamin B_{12} in November 2008. She described a significant history of fatigue, unrefreshing sleep, and widespread muscular pain that began almost three decades ago. Although she was formally diagnosed with fibromyalgia syndrome, her presentation reflected chronic fatigue syndrome. Within twenty-four hours of the first B_{12} injection, she noticed a marked improvement in her energy level and a lessening of her anxiety symptoms. This patient was taught how to self-inject vitamin B_{12} (3,000 micrograms of hydroxocobalamin) and was instructed to do the injections 2–3 times each week. As of May 2009, she reported feeling approximately 60–70 percent better overall. She was also contemplating a return to the workplace, something that she had not done for three years.

These two cases highlight the incredible therapeutic value that vitamin B_{12} has when it is administered by injection, given at the proper (most effective) dose, and injected frequently at regular intervals. It is also extremely cheap and cost-effective, and allows people to develop more self reliance and less dependence on their clinicians and the medical system as a whole.

TREATING RED BLOOD CELL ABNORMALITIES AND OXIDATIVE STRESS

OLIGOANTIGENIC (ELIMINATION) DIET

THERAPEUTIC EFFECT: To identify and reduce dietary intolerances (food allergies)

DAILY DOSAGE: Follow a diet that does not contain any implicated dietary items, or a rotation diet in which the allergenic foods are ingested infrequently

VITAMIN B_{12}

THERAPEUTIC EFFECT: Stops oxidative damage to the RBC membranes

DAILY DOSAGE: 1,000–5,000 micrograms hydroxocobalamin, tailored to the individual's needs; usually given weekly, several times each week, or more frequently

VITAMIN C

THERAPEUTIC EFFECT: Its antioxidant effects might return the abnormally shaped RBCs to normal

DAILY DOSAGE: 1–12 grams

VITAMIN E

THERAPEUTIC EFFECT: Antioxidant protects the RBCs from oxidative damage

DAILY DOSAGE: 400–1,200 IU (about 267–800 mg) of D-alpha tocopherol

POLYUNSATURATED OILS (EVENING PRIMROSE OIL OR FISH OIL)

THERAPEUTIC EFFECT: Both evening primrose oil and fish oil improve the function of RBCs

DAILY DOSAGE: 4,000 mg of evening primrose oil; or 1,500 mg of EPA and 500 mg of DHA (dosages may be increased)

GLUTATHIONE

THERAPEUTIC EFFECT: Maintains glutathione levels within the RBCs and has powerful antioxidant effects

DAILY DOSAGE: 1.0–1.5 teaspoons (approximately 420–600 mg) of liposomal glutathione

ALPHA-LIPOIC ACID (ALA)

THERAPEUTIC EFFECT: Indirectly raises glutathione levels and helps to recycle vitamins C and E

DAILY DOSAGE: 150–300 mg

GINKGO BILOBA EXTRACT

THERAPEUTIC EFFECT: Possesses biological properties that positively influence the function of RBCs

DAILY DOSAGE: 60–240 mg

VINPOCETINE

THERAPEUTIC EFFECT: Possesses significant antioxidant properties that limit oxidative damage to RBCs; also improves capillary blood flow

DAILY DOSAGE: 10 mg three times daily

GABA

THERAPEUTIC EFFECT: Reduces anxiety (and the output of catecholamines) with therapeutic effects similar to benzodiazepines

DAILY DOSAGE: 300–600 mg

GLYCINE

THERAPEUTIC EFFECT: Reduces anxiety (and the output of catecholamines) with therapeutic effects similar to benzodiazepines

DAILY DOSAGE: 5–40 grams mixed in juice and taken between meals

VITAMIN B_3

THERAPEUTIC EFFECT: Alleviates anxiety (and the output of catecholamines) by stimulating GABA receptors

DAILY DOSAGE: 2,000–4,500 mg of niacinamide (nicotinamide)

5-HTP

THERAPEUTIC EFFECT: Reduces anxiety (and the output of catecholamines) by increasing serotonin in the brain

DAILY DOSAGE: 200–900 mg

Summary

Abnormally shaped red blood cells and the resultant impairment in microcirculation underlie many of the clinical features of chronic fatigue syndrome. While it is apparent that CFS sufferers are under an excessive amount of oxidative stress, we still do not know the precise reasons for the abnormal RBCs. However, the increased oxidative stress points to many promising vitamin and other natural solutions aimed at "normalizing" the shape of the blood cells and improving quality of life for those with chronic fatigue.

CONCLUSION

Create an Individualized Treatment Plan

If you have chronic fatigue syndrome (CFS) and want to obtain a better and more enjoyable quality of life, it is important that the recommendations in this book are used in conjunction with a comprehensive holistic treatment plan, which includes lifestyle and dietary modifications, along with the vitamin and other treatments. To help you prioritize your symptoms and then implement treatments, I have created a step-by-step approach—the Prousky Plan—to assist you. This approach has been successfully used with many of my CFS patients. It should allow you to more effectively and precisely treat your own symptoms and overcome chronic fatigue.

The Prousky Plan

Step One: Incorporate many of the suggestions in Chapter 2: Lifestyle Modifications. These will help you create a more balanced life, and teach you to "pace" yourself in your daily activities. Pay special attention to the type and intensity of regular exercise and look for ways to make your home more ergonomically sound.

Step Two: Consider the treatments outlined in Chapter 3: Treating Allergies. Most people with CFS have chronic allergies and suffer from disabling gastrointestinal complaints, such as gas and bloating, constipation alternating with diarrhea, or adverse reactions to foods. Following these recommendations on eliminating allergies should substantially increase your quality of life and eliminate many chronic nuisance symptoms.

Step Three: Adopt the strategies described in Chapter 9: Treating Red Blood Cell Abnormalities and Oxidative Stress. I firmly believe that abnormal red blood cell (RBC) shape changes cause many of the clinical features of chronic fatigue. The scientific data on RBC abnormalities strongly supports the notion that chronic fatigue has an organic basis. The principal cause of these abnormalities is too much oxidative stress. I have seen many patients significantly improve from using a combination of the treatments described in this chapter.

Step Four: Add additional treatments to address the dominant symptoms of your chronic fatigue.

- If your dominant symptoms lead you to feel dizzy much of the time, especially when changing your posture, or if you have apparent cognitive problems, such as difficulty remembering things and concentrating, look at the treatments outlined in Chapter 4: Optimizing Autonomic and Central Nervous System Function.
- If your dominant symptoms involve adverse reactions to chemicals and heightened sensitivities to smells, and if the onset of your illness occurred around some type of toxic exposure, adopt the suggestions outlined in Chapter 5: A Detoxification Program for Chronic Fatigue.
- If your dominant symptoms include persistent cold and flu-like symptoms, and you always have a tendency to "catch" whatever is going around, look for answers in Chapter 6: Restoring Balance to the Immune System.
- If your dominant symptoms involve mental health disturbances, such as depression and anxiety, that never seem to get better, try the treatments outlined in Chapter 7: Treating Mental Health Problems.

- If your dominant symptoms include chronic muscle pain and even muscle weakness, adopt the strategies outlined in Chapter 8: Alleviating Muscular Dysfunction.

Step Five: When following these steps, do not adopt treatments from all of the chapters mentioned in Step Four. Pick the one chapter from the list that seems most appropriate for your situation and combine these new strategies to the treatments recommended in the first three steps. Then, give yourself at least 6–8 weeks before making any additional treatment changes. If after this time none of the treatments helped, then try a new set of options from another chapter in Step Four. If the treatments have helped after 6–8 weeks, continue them for another 3–6 months to see if your condition can be further stabilized. Most of the time, chronic fatigue can be adequately stabilized once an effective treatment plan is implemented. As more time passes, the condition usually becomes very manageable and less apt to impair your quality of life.

If you follow this plan, I believe you will avoid the need to take more mainstream medications. The program outlined in this book is designed to be practical, easy-to-follow, and very affordable. With the help of your clinician, I am confident that this comprehensive, holistic treatment plan will significantly improve your life and your health.

In the meantime, I am asking chronic fatigue sufferers (and their clinicians) who have utilized these recommendations to submit their results to me. I hope to include some of these clinical reports, along with the results of further research and scientific publications, in future editions. Correspondence can be sent by e-mail or regular mail to:

Jonathan E. Prousky, M.Sc., N.D.
Canadian College of Naturopathic Medicine
1255 Sheppard Avenue East
North York, Ontario, Canada M2K 1E2
E-mail: jprousky@ccnm.edu
Tel: 416-498-1255, ext. 235; Fax: 416-498-1611

RESOURCES

Several types of resources are listed to further assist you in obtaining more information. I have purposely kept this resource list to a minimum. Choosing the right books, websites, and health-care providers is a very personal decision, and ultimately it is up to you to find the most appropriate resources to suit your needs.

Because website addresses change frequently, the best approach may be to simply use an Internet search engine to find credible resources. When evaluating resources, it is important to ask several questions before accepting the information presented to you:

- Is the resource new or has it existed for many years? Resources with many years of operation are typically better and more reliable than ones having only a few years.

- Is the resource affiliated with an established educational institution? If so, this is a good sign since the resource probably has credibility.

- Is the resource comprehensive and inclusive of many different types of medical approaches (for example, advocates for both mainstream and complementary treatments), as opposed to subscribing to a singular approach only?

Adhering to these simple questions will help you find useful and reliable information.

Books

Bested, A.C., A.C. Logan, R. Howe. *Hope and Help for Chronic Fatigue Syndrome and Fibromyalgia,* 2nd edition. Nashville, TN: Cumberland House, 2008.

This book is designed to educate people suffering from chronic fatigue and fibromyalgia about their illnesses and to teach them coping skills that will improve their quality of life. Some of the issues covered in this book include understanding the symptoms and how diagnoses are made; causes of CFS; the role of stress and how to manage it; the therapeutic potential of medications, nutrition, and lifestyle changes; and legal issues.

Murray, M.T. *Chronic Fatigue Syndrome: How You Can Benefit from Diet, Vitamins, Minerals, Herbs, Exercise, and Other Natural Methods.* Rocklin, CA: Prima Health, 1994.

Offers clear and concise explanations of specific measures (detoxification, nutritional support, and adrenal balance) that can be taken to improve stamina, mental energy, and physical abilities. This book helps patients take control of their healing process using a completely natural approach.

Teitelbaum, J. *From Fatigued to Fantastic!* 3rd edition. New York: Penguin, 2007.

Jacob Teitelbaum's integrated treatment program is based on the clinically proven results of his landmark study and on his more than thirty years of experience in working with patients to overcome their illnesses. Using the most current information, Dr. Teitelbaum helps his readers evaluate their symptoms and develop an individualized program to eliminate them.

Journals

Journal of Chronic Fatigue Syndrome

www.cfs-news.org/jcfs.htm

This journal is an important forum for ongoing debates and discussions on issues related to chronic fatigue. It offers multidisciplinary original research, practical clinical management, case reports, and literature reviews intended for primary care physicians, psychologists, and specialists, as well as researchers studying this complex illness.

The CFIDS Chronicle • www.cfids.org/archives/

The CFIDS Chronicle is widely regarded as the most comprehensive print publication available on chronic fatigue syndrome. It contains treatment articles, coping tips, public policy and media reports, personal stories, and other information vital to people living with CFS.

Websites

CFIDS Association of America • www.cfids.org

The CFIDS Association of America is the largest and most active charitable organization dedicated to chronic fatigue syndrome (also known as chronic fatigue and immune dysfunction syndrome or CFIDS). Since 1987, the Association has invested more than $25 million in initiatives to bring an end to the pain, disability, and suffering caused by chronic fatigue.

Co-Cure ME/CFS and Fibromyalgia • www.co-cure.org

Begun in 1996, the Co-Cure (Cooperate and Communicate for a Cure) Project is a purely volunteer, patient-driven effort to promote the sharing of information about chronic fatigue syndrome and fibromyalgia and related disorders.

Jacob Teitelbaum, M.D. • www.jacobteitelbaum.com

Jacob Teitelbaum, M.D., and his team want to make the effective treatment of chronic fatigue and fibromyalgia available to as many people as possible. They accomplish this by providing those who suffer from CFS and fibromyalgia the tools they need to heal themselves, including an effective treatment protocol; teaching tools to make this information easily available; scientific research and studies; and help in finding physicians who specialize in treating CFS and fibromyalgia.

National ME/FM Action Network • www.mefmaction.net

The National ME/FM Action Network is a nonprofit organization founded in 1993. They are actively involved in issues that affect individuals who have myalgic encephalomyelitis, chronic fatigue syndrome, and fibromyalgia syndrome. They assist their membership through education, advocacy, support, and research.

Health-Care Provider Organizations

American Holistic Medical Association (AHMA)
www.holisticmedicine.org
The AHMA was founded in 1978 to unite licensed physicians who practice holistic medicine. It is the oldest holistic medicine organization of its kind and continues to strive toward creating collaboration among practitioners and those they work with, bringing an understanding of how the mind, body, and spirit all have a part in healing.

International Society for Orthomolecular Medicine (ISOM)
www.orthomed.org/ISOM/isom.html
The purpose of ISOM is to further the advancement of orthomolecular medicine throughout the world, to raise awareness of this rapidly growing and cost-effective practice of health care, and to unite the various groups already operating in this field. It educates health professionals and the public about orthomolecular medicine through publications, conferences, and seminars.

American Association of Naturopathic Physicians (AANP)
www.naturopathic.org
Founded in 1985, AANP is the national professional society representing licensed (or licensable) naturopathic physicians who have fulfilled a four-year, residential graduate program. Membership consists of more than 2,000 students, physicians, and supporting and corporate members who collectively strive to expand access to naturopathic medicine nationwide.

Canadian Association of Naturopathic Doctors (CAND)
www.cand.ca
CAND has been the national voice of the Canadian naturopathic profession since 1955, with a membership of over 1,500 naturopathic doctors and naturopathic medical students. It promotes naturopathic medicine to the public, corporations, insurance companies, and the federal government.

References

Chapter 1: What Is Chronic Fatigue Syndrome?

1. *Defining Moments: 20 Years of Making CFS History.* Charlotte, NC: CFIDS Association of America, 2008, pp. 4–5.

2. Leonard, J.A., S.R. Torres-Harding, M.G. Njoku. "The Face of CFS in the U.S." *The CFIDS Chronicle* (2005–2006): 16–21.

3. Donoghue, P.J., and M.E. Siegel. *Sick and Tired of Feeling Sick and Tired.* New York: W.W. Norton, 2000, p. 7.

4. Leonard, J.A., S.R. Torres-Harding, M.G. Njoku. "The Face of CFS in the U.S." *The CFIDS Chronicle* (2005–2006): 16–21.

5. Ibid.

6. Adapted from: Cornuz, J., I. Guessous, B. Favrat. "Fatigue: A Practical Approach to Diagnosis in Primary Care." *Can Med Assoc J* 174 (2006): 765–767. Craig, T., and S. Kakumanu. "Chronic Fatigue Syndrome: Evaluation and Treatment." *Am Fam Physician* 65 (2002): 1083–1090, 1095.

7. Okkes, I.M., S.K. Oskam, H. Lamberts. "The Probability of Specific Diagnoses for Patients Presenting with Common Symptoms to Dutch Family Physicians." *J Fam Pract* 51 (2002): 31–39.

8. Cornuz, J., I. Guessous, B. Favrat. "Fatigue: A Practical Approach to Diagnosis in Primary Care." *Can Med Assoc J* 174 (2006): 765–767.

9. Cornuz, J., I. Guessous, B. Favrat. "Fatigue: A Practical Approach to Diagnosis in Primary Care." *Can Med Assoc J* 174 (2006): 765–767. U.S. Department of Health and Human Services, Centers for Disease Control and Prevention. "CFS Toolkit for Health Care Professionals: Diagnosing CFS." (December 2008). Available online at: http://www.cdc.gov/CFS/pdf/Diagnosing_CFS.pdf.

10. Cornuz, J., I. Guessous, B. Favrat. "Fatigue: A Practical Approach to Diagnosis in Primary Care." *Can Med Assoc J* 174 (2006): 765–767.

11. U.S. Department of Health and Human Services, Centers for Disease Control and Prevention. "CFS Toolkit for Health Care Professionals: Diagnosing CFS." (December 2008). Available online at: http://www.cdc.gov/CFS/pdf/Diagnosing_CFS.pdf.

12. Dunstan, R.H., N.R. McGregor, H.L. Butt, et al. "Biochemical and Microbiological Anomalies in Chronic Fatigue Syndrome: The Development of Laboratory-based Tests and the Possible Role of Toxic Chemicals." *J Nutr Environ Med* 9 (1999): 97–108.

13. Wright, J.B., and D.W. Beverley. "Chronic Fatigue Syndrome." *Arch Dis Child* 79 (1998): 368–374.

14. Craig, T., and S. Kakumanu. "Chronic Fatigue Syndrome: Evaluation and Treatment." *Am Fam Physician* 65 (2002): 1083–1090, 1095.

15. Conti, F., L. Magrini, R. Priori, et al. "Eosinophil Cationic Protein Serum Levels and Allergy in Chronic Fatigue Syndrome." *Allergy* 51 (1996): 124–127.

16. Repka-Ramirez, M.S., K. Naranch, Y.J. Park, et al. "IgE Levels Are the Same in Chronic Fatigue Syndrome (CFS) and Control Subjects When Stratified by Allergy Skin Test Results and Rhinitis Types." *Ann Allergy Asthma Immunol* 87 (2001): 218–221.

17. Baraniuk, J.N., D.J. Clauw, E. Gaumond. "Rhinitis Symptoms in Chronic Fatigue Syndrome." *Ann Allergy Asthma Immunol* 81 (1998): 359–365.

18. Loblay, R.H., and A.R. Swain. "The Role of Food Intolerance in Chronic Fatigue Syndrome." In Hyde, B.M. (ed.). *Clinical and Scientific Basis of Myalgic Encephalomyelitis/Chronic Fatigue Syndrome.* Ottawa, ON, Canada: Nightingale Research Foundation, 1992, pp. 521–538.

19. Ferré Ybarz, L., V. Cardona Dahl, A. Cadahía García, et al. "Prevalence of Atopy in Chronic Fatigue Syndrome." [Spanish.] *Allergol Immunopathol (Madr)* 33 (2005): 42–47.

20. Loblay, R.H., and A.R. Swain. "The Role of Food Intolerance in Chronic Fatigue Syndrome." In Hyde, B.M. (ed.). *Clinical and Scientific Basis of Myalgic Encephalomyelitis/Chronic Fatigue Syndrome.* Ottawa, ON, Canada: Nightingale Research Foundation, 1992, pp. 521–538.

21. Craig, T., and S. Kakumanu. "Chronic Fatigue Syndrome: Evaluation and Treatment." *Am Fam Physician* 65 (2002): 1083–1090, 1095.

22. Rowe, P.C., and H. Calkins. "Neurally Mediated Hypotension and Chronic Fatigue Syndrome." *Am J Med* 105 (1998): 15S–21S. Schondorf, R., and R. Freeman. "The Importance of Orthostatic Intolerance in the Chronic Fatigue Syndrome." *Am J Med Sci* 317 (1999): 117–123. Schondorf, R., J. Benoit, T. Wein, et al. "Orthostatic Intolerance in the Chronic Fatigue Syndrome." *J Autonom Nerv Sys* 75 (1999): 192–201. Winkler, A.S., D. Blair, J.T. Marsden, et al. "Autonomic Function and Serum Erythropoietin Levels in Chronic Fatigue Syndrome." *J Psychosom Res* 56 (2004): 179–183. Freeman, R., and

A.L. Komaroff. "Does the Chronic Fatigue Syndrome Involve the Autonomic Nervous System?" *Am J Med* 102 (1997): 357–364. Karas, B., B.P. Grubb, K. Boehm, et al. "The Postural Orthostatic Tachycardia Syndrome: A Potentially Treatable Cause of Chronic Fatigue, Exercise Intolerance, and Cognitive Impairment in Adolescents." *PACE* 23 (2000): 344–351. LaManca, J.J., A. Peckerman, J. Walker, et al. "Cardiovascular Response During Head-up Tilt in Chronic Fatigue Syndrome." *Clin Physiol* 19 (1999): 111–120. De Becker, P., P. Dendale, K. De Meirleir, et al. "Autonomic Testing in Patients with Chronic Fatigue Syndrome." *Am J Med* 105 (1998): 22S–26S. Yoshiuchi, K., K.S. Quigley, K. Ohashi, et al. "Use of Time-frequency Analysis to Investigate Temporal Patterns of Cardiac Autonomic Response During Head-up Tilt in Chronic Fatigue Syndrome." *Autonom Neurosci* 113 (2004): 55–62. Yamamoto, Y., J.J. LaManca, B.H. Natelson. "A Measure of Heart Rate Variability Is Sensitive to Orthostatic Challenge in Women with Chronic Fatigue Syndrome." *Exp Biol Med* 228 (2003): 167–174. Pagani, M., and D. Lucini. "Chronic Fatigue Syndrome: A Hypothesis Focusing on the Autonomic Nervous System." *Clin Sci* 96 (1999): 117–125. Stewart, J., A. Weldon, N. Arlievsky, et al. "Neurally Mediated Hypotension and Autonomic Dysfunction Measured by Heart Rate Variability During Head-up Tilt Testing in Children with Chronic Fatigue Syndrome." *Clin Auton Res* 8 (1998): 221–230. Timmers, H.J., W. Wieling, P.M. Soetekouw, et al. "Hemodynamic and Neurohumoral Responses to Head-up Tilt in Patients with Chronic Fatigue Syndrome." *Clin Auton Res* 12 (2002): 273–280. Peckerman, A., J.J. La Manca, K.A. Krishna, et al. "Abnormal Impedance Cardiography Predicts Symptom Severity in Chronic Fatigue Syndrome." *Am J Med Sci* 326 (2003): 55–60. Stewart, J.M. "Autonomic Nervous System Dysfunction in Adolescents with Postural Orthostatic Tachycardia Syndrome and Chronic Fatigue Syndrome Is Characterized by Attenuated Vagal Baroreflex and Potentiated Sympathetic Vasomotion." *Pediatr Res* 48 (2000): 218–226.

23. Soetekouw, P.M., J.W. Lenders, G. Bleijenberg, et al. "Autonomic Function in Patients with Chronic Fatigue Syndrome." *Clin Auton Res* 9 (1999): 334–340. Timmers, H.J., W. Wieling, P.M. Soetekouw, et al. "Hemodynamic and Neurohumoral Responses to Head-up Tilt in Patients with Chronic Fatigue Syndrome." *Clin Auton Res* 12 (2002): 273–280.

24. Lange, G., S. Wang, J. DeLuca, et al. "Neuroimaging in Chronic Fatigue Syndrome." *Am J Med* 105 (1998): S50–S53.

25. Costa, D.C., C. Tannock, J. Brostoff. "Brainstem Perfusion Is Impaired in Chronic Fatigue Syndrome." *Q J Med* 88 (1995): 767–773.

26. Tirelli, U., F. Chierichetti, M. Tavio, et al. "Brain Positron Emission Tomography (PET) in Chronic Fatigue Syndrome." *Am J Med* 105 (1998): S54–S58.

27. Yoshiuchi, K., J. Farkas, B.H. Natelson. "Patients with Chronic Fatigue Syndrome Have Reduced Absolute Cortical Blood Flow." *Clin Physiol Funct Imaging* 26 (2006): 83–86.

28. Lane, R.J.M. "Neurological Features of Myalgic Encephalomyelitis." In Hyde, B.M. (ed.). *Clinical and Scientific Basis of Myalgic Encephalomyelitis/Chronic Fatigue Syndrome.* Ottawa, ON, Canada: Nightingale Research Foundation, 1992, pp. 395–399.

29. Anyanwu, E., A.W. Campbell, J. Jones. "The Neurological Significance of Abnormal Natural Killer Cell Activity in Chronic Toxigenic Mold Exposures." *Scientific World Journal* 3 (2003): 1128–1137. Sorenson, W.G. "Fungal Spores: Hazardous to Health?" *Environ Health Perspect* 107:Suppl 3 (1999): 469–472.

30. Australian Government, Department of the Environment, Water, Heritage, and the Arts. "Organochlorine Pesticides." (Accessed January 2009). Available online at: www.environment.gov.au/settlements/chemicals/scheduled-waste/ocp.html.

31. Katz, K.D., D.E. Brooks, M.C. Furtado, et al. "Toxicity, Organophosphate." eMedicine, WebMD. (Accessed January 2009). Available online at: www.emedicine.medscape.com/article/167726-overview.

32. Dunstan, R.H., M. Donohoe, W. Taylor, et al. "A Preliminary Investigation of Chlorinated Hydrocarbons and Chronic Fatigue Syndrome." *Med J Aust* 163 (1995): 294–297.

33. Dunstan, R.H., T.K. Roberts, M. Donohoe, et al. "Bioaccumulated Chlorinated Hydrocarbons and Red/white Blood Cell Parameters." *Biochem Molec Med* 58 (1996): 77–84.

34. Behan, P.O. "Chronic Fatigue Syndrome as a Delayed Reaction to Chronic Low-dose Organophosphate Exposure." *J Nutr Environ Med* 6 (1996): 341–350.

35. Racciatti, D., J. Vecchiet, A. Ceccomancini, et al. "Chronic Fatigue Syndrome Following a Toxic Exposure." *Sci Total Environ* 270 (2001): 27–31.

36. See, D.M., and J.G. Tilles. "Alpha-interferon Treatment of Patients with Chronic Fatigue Syndrome." *Immunol Invest* 25 (1996): 153–164. Dillman, R.O. "The Clinical Experience with Interleukin-2 in Cancer Therapy." *Cancer Biother* 9 (1994): 183–209.

37. Ojo-Amaize, E.A., E.J. Conley, J.B. Peter. "Decreased Natural Killer Cell Activity Is Associated with Severity of Chronic Fatigue Immune Dysfunction Syndrome." *Clin Infect Dis* 18 (1994): S157–S159. Whiteside, T.L., and D. Friberg. "Natural Killer Cells and Natural Killer Cell Activity in Chronic Fatigue Syndrome." *Am J Med* 105 (1998): S27–S34.

38. Craig, T., and S. Kakumanu. "Chronic Fatigue Syndrome: Evaluation and Treatment." *Am Fam Physician* 65 (2002): 1083–1090, 1095. Werbach, M.R. "Chronic Fatigue Syndrome: How Far Have We Come?" *J Nutr Environ Med* 10 (2000): 181–188.

39. Evengard, B., R.S. Schacterle, A.L. Komaroff. "Chronic Fatigue Syndrome: New Insights and Old Ignorance." *J Intern Med* 246 (1999): 455–469.

40. Craig, T., and S. Kakumanu. "Chronic Fatigue Syndrome: Evaluation and

Treatment." *Am Fam Physician* 65 (2002): 1083–1090, 1095. Werbach, M.R. "Chronic Fatigue Syndrome: How Far Have We Come?" *J Nutr Environ Med* 10 (2000): 181–188.

41. Galland, L., M. Lee, H. Bueno, et al. "*Giardia lamblia* Infection as a Cause of Chronic Fatigue." *J Nutr Med* 1 (1990): 27–31.

42. Craig, T., and S. Kakumanu. "Chronic Fatigue Syndrome: Evaluation and Treatment." *Am Fam Physician* 65 (2002): 1083–1090, 1095.

43. Wearden, A.J., and L. Appleby. "Research on Cognitive Complaints and Cognitive Functioning in Patients with Chronic Fatigue Syndrome (CFS): What Conclusions Can We Draw?" *J Psychosom Res* 41 (1996): 197–211.

44. Wearden, A.J., and L. Appleby. "Research on Cognitive Complaints and Cognitive Functioning in Patients with Chronic Fatigue Syndrome (CFS): What Conclusions Can We Draw?" *J Psychosom Res* 41 (1996): 197–211. McCluskey, D.R. "Chronic Fatigue Syndrome: Its Cause and a Strategy for Management." *Compr Ther* 24 (1998): 357–363.

45. Ibid.

46. Griffith, J.P., and F.A. Zarrouf. "A Systematic Review of Chronic Fatigue Syndrome: Don't Assume It's Depression." *Prim Care Companion J Clin Psychiatry* 10 (2008): 120–128.

47. Riley, M.S., C.J. O'Brien, D.R. McCluskey, et al. "Aerobic Work Capacity in Patients with Chronic Fatigue Syndrome." *Br Med J* 301 (1990): 953–956.

48. LaManca, J.J., S.A. Sisto, J. DeLuca, et al. "Influence of Exhaustive Treadmill Exercise on Cognitive Functioning in Chronic Fatigue Syndrome." *Am J Med* 105 (1998): S59–S65. Blackwood, S.K., S.M. MacHale, M.J. Power, et al. "Effects of Exercise on Cognitive and Motor Function in Chronic Fatigue Syndrome and Depression." *J Neurol Neurosurg Psychiatry* 65 (1998): 541–546.

49. Wallace, D.J., S. Shapiro, R.S. Panush. "Update of Fibromyalgia Syndrome." *Bull Rheum Dis* 48:5 (1999): 1–4.

50. Klein, R., and P.A. Berg. "High Incidence of Antibodies to 5-Hydroxytryptamine, Gangliosides and Phospholipids in Patients with Chronic Fatigue and Fibromyalgia Syndrome and Their Relatives: Evidence for a Clinical Entity of Both Disorders." *Eur J Med Res* 1 (1995): 21–26.

51. Fulle, S., P. Mecocci, G. Fano, et al. "Specific Oxidative Alterations in Vastus Lateralis Muscle of Patients with the Diagnosis of Chronic Fatigue Syndrome." *Free Radic Biol Med* 29 (2000): 1252–1259.

52. Pall, M.L. "Cobalamin Used in Chronic Fatigue Syndrome Therapy Is a Nitric Oxide Scavenger." *J Chronic Fatigue Syndr* 8 (2001): 39–44. Pall, M.L, and J.D. Satterlee. "Elevated Nitric Oxide/Peroxynitrite Mechanism for the Common Etiology of Multiple Chemical Sensitivity, Chronic Fatigue Syndrome, and Post-traumatic Stress Disorder." *Ann N Y Acad Sci* 933 (2001): 323–329.

53. Pall, M.L. "NMDA Sensitization and Stimulation by Peroxynitrite, Nitric Oxide, and Organic Solvents as the Mechanism of Chemical Sensitivity in Multiple Chemical Sensitivity." *FASEB J* 16 (2002): 1407–1417. Pall, M.L. "Elevated Nitric Oxide/Peroxynitrite Theory of Multiple Chemical Sensitivity: Central Role of N-Methyl-D-Aspartate Receptors in the Sensitivity Mechanism." *Environ Health Perspect* 111 (2003): 1461–1464.

54. Manuel Keenoy, B., G. Moorkens, J. Vertommen, et al. "Antioxidant Status and Lipoprotein Peroxidation in Chronic Fatigue Syndrome." *Life Sci* 68 (2001): 2037–2049. Richards, R.S., T.K. Roberts, N.R. McGregor, et al. "Blood Parameters Indicative of Oxidative Stress Are Associated with Symptom Expression in Chronic Fatigue Syndrome." *Redox Rep* 5 (2000): 35–41.

55. Logan, A.L., and C. Wong. "Chronic Fatigue Syndrome: Oxidative Stress and Dietary Modifications." *Altern Med Rev* 6 (2001): 450–459.

56. Simpson, L.O., B.I. Shand, R.J. Olds. "Blood Rheology and Myalgic Encephalomyelitis: A Pilot Study." *Pathology* 18 (1986): 190–192.

57. Simpson, L.O. "Nondiscocytic Erythrocytes in Myalgic Encephalomyelitis." *N Z Med J* 102 (1989): 126–127.

Chapter 2: Lifestyle Modifications

1. Paterson, E.T. "Staged Management for Chronic Fatigue Syndrome." *J Orthomolecular Med* 10 (1995): 70–78.

2. Carruthers, B.M., A.K. Jain, K.L. De Meirleir, et al. "Myalgic Encephalomyelitis/Chronic Fatigue Syndrome: Clinical Working Case Definition, Diagnostic and Treatment Protocols." *J Chronic Fatigue Syndr* 11 (2003): 7–115.

3. Paterson, E.T. "Staged Management for Chronic Fatigue Syndrome." *J Orthomolecular Med* 10 (1995): 70–78. Carruthers, B.M., A.K. Jain, K.L. De Meirleir, et al. "Myalgic Encephalomyelitis/Chronic Fatigue Syndrome: Clinical Working Case Definition, Diagnostic and Treatment Protocols." *J Chronic Fatigue Syndr* 11 (2003): 7–115.

4. Carruthers, B.M., A.K. Jain, K.L. De Meirleir, et al. "Myalgic Encephalomyelitis/Chronic Fatigue Syndrome: Clinical Working Case Definition, Diagnostic and Treatment Protocols." *J Chronic Fatigue Syndr* 11 (2003): 7–115.

Chapter 3: Treating Allergies

1. Bellanti, J.A., A. Sabra, H.J. Castro, et al. "Are Attention Deficit Hyperactivity Disorder and Chronic Fatigue Syndrome Allergy Related? What is Fibromyalgia?" *Allergy Asthma Proc* 26 (2005): 19–28.

2. Nisenbaum, R., M. Reyes, A. Jones, et al. "Course of Illness among Patients with Chronic Fatigue Syndrome in Wichita, Kansas." [Abstract #49.] Paper presented at the American Association for Chronic Fatigue Syndrome conference, Seattle, WA, January 2001.

3. Jacobsen, M.B., P. Aukrust, E. Kittang, et al. "Relation between Food Provocation and Systemic Immune Activation in Patients with Food Intolerance." *Lancet* 356 (2000): 400–401.

4. Emms, T.M., T.K. Robers, H.L. Butt, et al. "Food Intolerance in Chronic Fatigue Syndrome." [Abstract #15.] Paper presented at the American Association for Chronic Fatigue Syndrome conference, Seattle, WA, January 2001.

5. Gomborone, J.E., D.A. Gorard, P.A Dewsnap, et al. "Prevalence of Irritable Bowel Syndrome in Chronic Fatigue." *J R Coll Physicians Lond* 30 (1996): 512–513. Aaron, L.A., M.M. Burke, D. Buchwald. "Overlapping Conditions among Patients with Chronic Fatigue Syndrome, Fibromyalgia, and Temporomandibular Disorder." *Arch Intern Med* 160 (2000): 221–227.

6. Borok, G. "Another Answer to Yuppie Flu?" *S Afr Med J* 76 (1989): 176.

7. Gaby, A.R. "The Role of Hidden Food Allergy/Intolerance in Chronic Disease." *Altern Med Rev* 3 (1998): 90–100.

8. Gibson, S.L., and R.G. Gibson. "A Multidimensional Treatment Plan for Chronic Fatigue Syndrome." *J Nutr Environ Med* 9 (1999): 47–54.

9. Komaroff, A.L., L.R. Fagioli, A.M. Geiger, et al. "An Examination of the Working Case Definition of Chronic Fatigue Syndrome." *Am J Med* 100 (1996): 56–64.

10. Victor, B.S., M. Lubetsky, J.F. Greden. "Somatic Manifestations of Caffeinism." *J Clin Psychiatry* 42 (1981): 185–188.

11. Greden, J.F., P. Fontaine, M. Lubetsky, et al. "Anxiety and Depression Associated with Caffeinism among Psychiatric Inpatients." *Am J Psychiatry* 135 (1978): 963–966.

12. Greden, J.F. "Anxiety or Caffeinism: A Diagnostic Dilemma." *Am J Psychiatry* 131 (1974): 1089–1092.

13. Alberti, K.G., and M. Nattress. "Lactic Acidosis." *Lancet* 2 (1977): 25–29.

14. Monteiro, M.G., M.A. Schuckit, M. Irwin. "Subjective Feelings of Anxiety in Young Men after Ethanol and Diazepam Infusions." *J Clin Psychiatry* 51 (1990): 12–16.

15. Roelofs, S.M. "Hyperventilation, Anxiety, Craving for Alcohol: A Subacute Alcohol Withdrawal Syndrome." *Alcohol* 2 (1985): 501–505.

16. Rainey, J.M., Jr., C.E. Frohman, R.R. Freedman, et al. "Specificity of Lactate Infusion as a Model of Anxiety." *Psychopharmacol Bull* 20 (1984): 45–49. Maddock, R.J., and J. Mateo-Bermudez. "Elevated Serum Lactate Following Hyperventilation During Glucose Infusion in Panic Disorder." *Biol Psychiatry* 27 (1990): 411–418. Maddock, R.J., C.S. Carter, D.W. Gietzen. "Elevated Serum Lactate Associated with Panic Attacks Induced by Hyperventilation." *Psychiatry Res* 38 (1991): 301–311.

17. Greenberg, D.B. "Neurasthenia in the 1980s: Chronic Mononucleosis,

Chronic Fatigue Syndrome, and Anxiety and Depressive Disorders." *Psychosomatics* 31 (1990): 129–137.

18. Gaby, A.R. "The Role of Hidden Food Allergy/Intolerance in Chronic Disease." *Altern Med Rev* 3 (1998): 90–100.

19. Mandell, M. "Cerebral Reactions in Allergenic Patients. Illustrative Case Histories and Comments." In Williams R.J., and D.K. Kalita (eds.). *A Physician's Handbook on Orthomolecular Medicine.* New Canaan, CT: Keats Publishing, 1977, 130–139.

20. Miller, A.L. "The Pathogenesis, Clinical Implications, and Treatment of Intestinal Hyperpermeability." *Altern Med Rev* 2 (1997): 330–345.

21. Peters, T.J., and I. Bjarnason. "Uses and Abuses of Intestinal Permeability Measurements." *Can J Gastroenterol* 2 (1988): 127–132.

22. Ventura, M.T., L. Polimeno, A.C. Amoruso, et al. "Intestinal Permeability in Patients with Adverse Reactions to Food." *Dig Liver Dis* 38 (2006): 732–736.

23. Miller, A.L. "The Pathogenesis, Clinical Implications, and Treatment of Intestinal Hyperpermeability." *Altern Med Rev* 2 (1997): 330–345.

24. Wong, C. "Leaky Gut Syndrome/Intestinal Permeability." About.com. (Accessed April 2008). Available online at: www.altmedicine.about.com/od/healthconditionsdisease/a/TestLeakyGut.htm.

25. Gaby, A.R. "The Role of Hidden Food Allergy/Intolerance in Chronic Disease." *Altern Med Rev* 3 (1998): 90–100. Egger, J. "Food Allergy and the Central Nervous System." In Schmidt, E. (ed.). *Food Allergy, Nestlé Nutrition Workshop Series, Volume 17.* New York: Vevey/Raven Press, 1988, pp. 159–175.

26. Egger, J. "Food Allergy and the Central Nervous System." In Schmidt, E. (ed.). *Food Allergy, Nestlé Nutrition Workshop Series, Volume 17.* New York: Vevey/Raven Press, 1988, pp. 159–175. Egger, J., J. Wilson, C.M. Carter, et al. "Is Migraine Food Allergy? A Double-blind Controlled Trial of Oligoantigenic Diet Treatment." *Lancet* 2 (1983): 865–869.

27. Egger, J., J. Wilson, C.M. Carter, et al. "Is Migraine Food Allergy? A Double-blind Controlled Trial of Oligoantigenic Diet Treatment." *Lancet* 2 (1983): 865–869.

28. Miller, A.L. "The Pathogenesis, Clinical Implications, and Treatment of Intestinal Hyperpermeability." *Altern Med Rev* 2 (1997): 330–345.

29. Tang, Z.F., Y.B. Ling, N. Lin, et al. "Glutamine and Recombinant Human Growth Hormone Protect Intestinal Barrier Function Following Portal Hypertension Surgery." *World J Gastroenterol* 13 (2007): 2223–2228. Lima, N.L., A.M. Soares, R.M. Mota, et al. "Wasting and Intestinal Barrier Function in Children Taking Alanyl-glutamine-Supplemented Enteral Formula." *J Pediatr Gastroenterol Nutr* 44 (2007): 365–374. Li, Y., Z. Yu, F. Liu, et al. "Oral Glu-

tamine Ameliorates Chemotherapy-induced Changes of Intestinal Permeability and Does Not Interfere with the Antitumor Effect of Chemotherapy in Patients with Breast Cancer: A Prospective Randomized Trial." *Tumori* 92 (2006): 396–401. van den Berg, A., W.P. Fetter, E.A. Westerbeek, et al. "The Effect of Glutamine-enriched Enteral Nutrition on Intestinal Permeability in Very-low-birth-weight Infants: A Randomized Controlled Trial." *JPEN J Parenter Enteral Nutr* 30 (2006): 408–414. Choi, K., S.S. Lee, S.J. Oh, et al. "The Effect of Oral Glutamine on 5-Fluorouracil/Leucovorin-induced Mucositis/Stomatitis Assessed by Intestinal Permeability Test." *Clin Nutr* 26 (2007): 57–62.

30. "L-Glutamine." *Altern Med Rev* 6 (2001): 406–410.

31. Heyman, M., K. Terpend, S. Ménard. "Effects of Specific Lactic Acid Bacteria on the Intestinal Permeability to Macromolecules and the Inflammatory Condition." *Acta Paediatr* Suppl 94 (2005): 34–36. Laitinen, K., and E. Isolauri. "Management of Food Allergy: Vitamins, Fatty Acids or Probiotics?" *Eur J Gastroenterol Hepatol* 17 (2005): 1305–1311.

32. Logan, A.C., A.V. Rao, D. Irani. "Chronic Fatigue Syndrome: Lactic Acid Bacteria May Be of Therapeutic Value." *Med Hypotheses* 60 (2003): 915–923.

33. Kajander, K., K. Hatakka, T. Poussa, et al. "A Probiotic Mixture Alleviates Symptoms in Irritable Bowel Syndrome Patients: A Controlled 6-Month Intervention." *Aliment Pharmacol Ther* 22 (2005): 387–394. Kim, H.J., M.I. Vazquez Roque, M. Camilleri, et al. "A Randomized Controlled Trial of a Probiotic Combination VSL# 3 and Placebo in Irritable Bowel Syndrome with Bloating." *Neurogastroenterol Motil* 17 (2005): 687–696. Whorwell, P.J., L. Altringer, J. Morel, et al. "Efficacy of an Encapsulated Probiotic *Bifidobacterium infantis* 35624 in Women with Irritable Bowel Syndrome." *Am J Gastroenterol* 101 (2006): 1581–1590. Guyonnet, D., O. Chassany, P. Ducrotte, et al. "Effect of a Fermented Milk Containing *Bifidobacterium animalis* DN-173 010 on the Health-related Quality of Life and Symptoms in Irritable Bowel Syndrome in Adults in Primary Care: A Multicentre, Randomized, Double-blind, Controlled Trial." *Aliment Pharmacol Ther* 26 (2007): 475–486.

34. Pearce, F.L., A.D. Befus, J. Bienenstock. "Mucosal Mast Cells. III. Effect of Quercetin and Other Flavonoids on Antigen-induced Histamine Secretion from Rat Intestinal Mast Cells." *J Allergy Clin Immunol* 73 (1984): 819–823.

35. Gugler, R., M. Leschik, H.J. Dengler. "Disposition of Quercetin in Man After Single Oral and Intravenous Doses." *Eur J Clin Pharmacol* 9 (1975): 229–234.

36. "Quercetin." *Altern Med Rev* 3 (1998): 140–143.

37. Luostarinen, L., T. Pirttila, P. Collin. "Coeliac Disease Presenting with Neurological Disorders." *Eur Neurol* 42 (1999): 132–135.

38. Logan, A.C., and C. Wong. "Chronic Fatigue Syndrome: Oxidative Stress and Dietary Modifications." *Altern Med Rev* 6 (2001): 450–459.

39. Skowera, A., M. Peakman, A. Cleare, et al. "High Prevalence of Serum Markers of Coeliac Disease in Patients with Chronic Fatigue Syndrome." *J Clin Pathol* 54 (2001): 335–336.

40. Pare, P., P. Douville, D. Caron, et al. "Adult Celiac Sprue: Changes in the Pattern of Clinical Recognition." *J Clin Gasteroenterol* 10 (1988): 395–400.

Chapter 4: Optimizing Autonomic and Central Nervous System Function

1. Heseker, H., W. Kubler, V. Pudel, et al. "Psychological Disorders as Early Symptoms of Mild-to-moderate Vitamin Deficiency." *Ann N Y Acad Sci* 669 (1992): 352–357.

2. Heap, L.C., T.J. Peters, S. Wessely. "Vitamin B Status in Patients with Chronic Fatigue Syndrome." *J R Soc Med* 92 (1999): 183–185.

3. Peres, M.F., E. Zukerman, W.B. Young, et al. "Fatigue in Chronic Migraine Patients." *Cephalgia* 22 (2002): 720–724.

4. Schoenen, J., M. Lenaerts, E. Bastings. "High-dose Riboflavin as a Prophylactic Treatment of Migraine: Results of an Open Pilot Study." *Cephalgia* 14 (1994): 328–329. Schoenen, J., J. Jacquy, M. Lenaerts. "Effectiveness of High-dose Riboflavin in Migraine Prophylaxis: A Randomized Controlled Trial." *Neurology* 50 (1998): 466–470. Boehnke, C., U. Reuter, U. Flach, et al. "High-dose Riboflavin Treatment Is Effective in Migraine Prophylaxis: An Open Study in a Tertiary Care Centre." *Euro J Neurol* 11 (2004): 475–477.

5. Schoenen, J., M. Lenaerts, E. Bastings. "High-dose Riboflavin as a Prophylactic Treatment of Migraine: Results of an Open Pilot Study." *Cephalgia* 14 (1994): 328–329.

6. Hoffer, A. "Vitamin B3 Dependency: Chronic Pellagra." *Townsend Letter for Doctors and Patients* 207 (2000): 66–73.

7. Forsyth, L.M., H.G. Preuss, A.L. MacDowell, et al. "Therapeutic Effects of Oral NADH on the Symptoms of Patients with Chronic Fatigue Syndrome." *Ann Allergy Asthma Immunol* 82 (1999): 185–191.

8. Forsyth, L.M.. A.L. MacDowell-Carnciro, G.D. Birkmayer, et al. "NADH: A New Therapeutic Approach in Chronic Fatigue Syndrome (CFS)." (March 2009). Available online at: www.enadh.com/case_physic.html.

9. Santaella, M.L., I. Font, O.M. Disdier. "Comparison of Oral Nicotinamide Adenine Dinucleotide (NADH) versus Conventional Therapy for Chronic Fatigue Syndrome." *P R Health Sci J* 23 (2004): 89–93.

10. Morrow, J.D., W.G. Parsons, 3rd., L.J. Roberts, 2nd. "Release of Markedly Increased Quantities of Prostaglandin D2 in Vivo in Humans Following the Administration of Nicotinic Acid." *Prostaglandins* 38 (1989): 263–274.

11. Prousky, J., and D. Seely. "The Treatment of Migraines and Tension-type

Headaches with Intravenous and Oral Niacin (Nicotinic Acid): Systematic Review of the Literature." *Nutr J* 4 (2005): 3.

12. Bicknell, F., and F. Prescott. *Vitamins in Medicine,* 3rd ed. Milwaukee, WI: Life Foundation for Nutritional Research, 1953, p. 346.

13. Sahai-Srivastava, S., R. Cowan, D.Y. Ko. "Pathophysiology and Treatment of Migraine and Related Headache." eMedicine, WebMD. (November 2007). Available online at: www.emedicine.com/neuro/topic517.htm.

14. Hall, J.A. "Enhancing Niacin's Effect for Migraine." *Cortlandt Forum* (July 1991): 46. Prousky, J., and E. Sykes. "Two Case Reports on the Treatment of Acute Migraine with Niacin. Its Hypothetical Mechanism of Action upon Calcitonin-gene Related Peptide and Platelets." *J Orthomolecular Med* 18 (2003): 108–110.

15. Dubey, A.K., P.R. Shankar, D. Upadhyaya,, et al. "*Ginkgo biloba*—An Appraisal." *Kathmandu Univ Med J (KUMJ)* 2 (2004): 225–229.

16. Ahlemeyer, B., and J. Krieglstein. "Neuroprotective Effects of *Ginkgo biloba* Extract." *Cell Mol Life Sci* 60 (2003): 1779–1792.

17. Miller, L.G., and B. Freeman. "Possible Subdural Hematoma Associated with *Ginkgo biloba.*" *J Herb Pharmacother* 2 (2002): 57–63.

18. Feher, G., K. Koltai, G. Kesmarky, et al. "Effect of Parenteral or Oral Vinpocetine on the Hemorheological Parameters of Patients with Chronic Cerebrovascular Diseases." *Phytomedicine* 16 (2009): 111–117.

19. "Vinpocetine. Monograph." *Altern Med Rev* 7 (2002): 240–243.

20. Baschetti, R. "Chronic Fatigue Syndrome and Licorice." (Letter.) *N Z Med J* 108 (1995): 156–157. Baschetti, R. "What Causes Chronic Fatigue?" *Can Med Assoc J* 160 (1999): 636.

21. Baschetti, R. "Chronic Fatigue Syndrome and Licorice." (Letter.) *N Z Med J* 108 (1995): 156–157.

22. Baschetti, R. "Chronic Fatigue Syndrome and Licorice." (Letter.) *N Z Med J* 108 (1995): 156–157. Baschetti, R. "What Causes Chronic Fatigue?" *Can Med Assoc J* 160 (1999): 636.

Chapter 5: A Detoxification Program for Chronic Fatigue

1. Liska, D.J. "The Detoxification Enzyme Systems." *Altern Med Rev* 3 (1998): 187–198.

2. Crinnion, W.J. "Environmental Medicine, Part 4: Pesticides—Biologically Persistent and Ubiquitous Toxins." *Altern Med Rev* 5 (2000): 432–447.

3. Schnare, D.W., G. Denk, M. Shields, et al. "Evaluation of a Detoxification Regimen for Fat-stored Xenobiotics." *Med Hypotheses* 9 (1982): 265–282. Schnare, D.W., M. Ben, M.G. Shields. "Body Burden Reductions of PCBs, PBBs and Chlorinated Pesticides in Human Subjects." *AMBIO* 13 (1984): 378–380.

Kilburn, K.H., R.H. Warsaw, M.G. Shields. "Neurobehavioral Dysfunction in Firemen Exposed to Polychlorinated Biphenyls (PCBs): Possible Improvement after Detoxification." *Arch Environ Health* 44 (1989): 345–350. Tretjak, Z., M. Shields, S.L. Beckmann. "PCB Reduction and Clinical Improvement by Detoxification: An Unexploited Approach?" *Human Exper Toxicol* 9 (1990): 235–244. Cecchini, M.A., D.E. Root, J.R. Rachunow, et al. "Chemical Exposures at the World Trade Center: Use of the Hubbard Sauna Detoxification Regimen to Improve the Health Status of the New York City Rescue Workers Exposed to Toxicants." *Townsend Letter for Doctors and Patients* 273 (2006): 58–65.

4. Pizzorno, J.E. "Detoxification: A Naturopathic Perspective." *Nat Med J* 1 (1998): 6–17.

5. Ibid.

6. Ibid.

7. Prousky, J. "Double Agent Niacin—Its Beneficial Effect upon the Lipid Profile, but Its Adverse Effect upon Plasma Homocysteine: A Case Report." *Queen's Health Sci J* 8 (2006): 34–38. Groff, J.L., S.S. Gropper, S.M. Hunt. *Advanced Nutrition and Human Metabolism,* 2nd Edition. St. Paul, MN: West Publishing, 1995, pp. 250–251.

8. Carlson, L.A., L. Orö, J. Ostman. "Effect of a Single Dose of Nicotinic Acid on Plasma Lipids in Patients with Hyperlipoproteinemia." *Acta Med Scand* 183 (1968): 457–465. Nye, E.R., and B. Buchanon. "Short-term Effect of Nicotinic Acid on Plasma Level and Turnover of Free Fatty Acids in Sheep and Man." *J Lipid Res* 10 (1969): 193–196.

9. Simopoulos, A.P. "Genetic Variation and Nutrition." *Nutr Rev* 57 (1999): S10–S19.

10. Ibid.

11. Bulow, J. "Adipose Tissue Blood Flow During Exercise." *Danish Med Bull* 30 (1983): 85–100.

12. Friedberg, S.J., W.R. Harlan, Jr., D.L. Trout, et al. "The Effect of Exercise on the Concentration and Turnover of Plasma Nonesterified Fatty Acids." *J Clin Invest* 39 (1960): 215. Carlson, L.A., and B. Pernow. "Studies on Blood Lipids During Exercise." *J Lab Clin Med* 58 (1961): 673–681. Friedberg, S.J., P.B. Sher, M.D. Bogdonoff, et al. "The Dynamics of Plasma Free Fatty Acid Metabolism During Exercise." *J Lipid Res* 4 (1963): 34–38. Horstman, D., J. Mendez, E.R. Buskirk, et al. "Lipid Metabolism During Heavy and Moderate Exercise." *Med Sci Sports* 3 (1971): 18–23. Taylor, A.W., D.W. Shoemann, R. Lovlin, et al. "Plasma Free Fatty Acid Mobilization with Graded Exercise." *J Sports Med* 11 (1971): 234–240. Wirth, A., G. Schlierf, G. Schetler. "Physical Activity and Lipid Metabolism." *Klin Wochenshr* 57 (1979): 1195.

13. Findlay, G.M., and A.S.W. de Freitas. "DDT Movement from Adipocyte to

Muscle Cell During Lipid Utilization." *Nature* 229 (1971): 63. de Freitas, A.S., and R.J. Norstrom. "Turnover and Metabolism of Polychlorinated Biphenyls in Relation to Their Chemical Structure and the Movement of Lipids in the Pigeon." *Can J Physiol Pharmacol* 52 (1974): 1081–1094. Mitjavila, S., G. Carrera, Y. Fernandez. "Evaluation of the Toxic Risk of Accumulated DDT in the Rat: During Fat Mobilization." *Arch Environ Contam Toxicol* 10 (1981): 471–481.

14. Davis, W. "Infrared Sauna Therapy: Improving Clinical Symptoms of Chemical Toxicity." *Naturopathic Doctor News and Review* 4:12 (2008): 15–17.

15. Pizzorno, J.E. "Detoxification: A Naturopathic Perspective." *Nat Med J* 1 (1998): 6–17.

16. Davis, W. "Infrared Sauna Therapy: Improving Clinical Symptoms of Chemical Toxicity." *Naturopathic Doctor News and Review* 4:12 (2008): 15–17.

17. Masuda, A., T. Kihara, T. Fukudome, et al. "The Effects of Repeated Thermal Therapy for Two Patients with Chronic Fatigue Syndrome." *J Psychosom Res* 58 (2005): 383–387.

18. Masuda, A., T. Munemoto, C. Tei. "A New Treatment: Thermal Therapy for Chronic Fatigue Syndrome." *Nippon Rinsho* 65 (2007): 1093–1098.

19. Davis, W. "Infrared Sauna Therapy: Improving Clinical Symptoms of Chemical Toxicity." *Naturopathic Doctor News and Review* 4:12 (2008): 15–17.

20. Ibid.

21. Shepherd, J., J.M. Stewart, J.G. Clark, et al. "Sequential Changes in Plasma Lipoproteins and Body Fat Composition During Polyunsaturated Fat Feeding in Man." *Br J Nutr* 44 (1980): 265–271.

22. Ibid.

23. Pizzorno, J.E. "Detoxification: A Naturopathic Perspective." *Nat Med J* 1 (1998): 6–17.

Chapter 6: Restoring Balance to the Immune System

1. Gaby, A.R. "Preventing Recurrent Infection." (Commentary.) *Nutrition and Healing* 4:11 (1997): 1, 10–11.

2. Ringsdorf, W.M., Jr., E. Cheraskin, R.R. Ramsay, Jr. "Sucrose, Neutrophilic Phagocytosis and Resistance to Disease." *Dent Surv* 52 (1976): 46–48.

3. Sanchez, A., J.L. Reeser, H.S. Lau, et al. "Role of Sugars in Human Neutrophilic Phagocytosis." *Am J Clin Nutr* 26 (1973): 1180–1184.

4. Horrigan, L.A., J.P. Kelly, T.J. Connor. "Immunomodulatory Effects of Caffeine: Friend or Foe?" *Pharmacol Ther* 111 (2006): 877–892.

5. Keusch, G.T. "Nutrition and Infection." In Shills, M.E., J.A. Olson, M. Shike (eds.). *Modern Nutrition in Health and Disease,* 8th Edition. Media, PA: Williams & Wilkins, 1994, pp. 1241–1258.

6. Shankar, A.H. "Nutritional Modulation of Immune Function and Infectious Disease." In Bowman, B.A., and R.M. Russell (eds.). *Present Knowledge in Nutrition,* 8th Edition. Washington, DC: ILSI Press, 2001, pp. 686–700.

7. Glasziou, P.P., and D.E. Mackerras. "Vitamin A Supplementation in Infectious Diseases: A Meta-analysis." *Br Med J* 306 (1993): 366–370.

8. Ronzio, R.A. "Nutritional Support for the Immune System." *Am J Nat Med* 5:3 (1998): 18–22.

9. Weeks, B.S. "Vitamin A and Beta-carotene." *J Orthomolecular Med* 18 (2003): 131–145.

10. Ibid.

11. Shankar, A.H. "Nutritional Modulation of Immune Function and Infectious Disease." In Bowman, B.A., and R.M. Russell (eds.). *Present Knowledge in Nutrition,* 8th Edition. Washington, DC: ILSI Press, 2001, pp. 686–700.

12. Ronzio, R.A. "Nutritional Support for the Immune System." *Am J Nat Med* 5:3 (1998): 18–22.

13. Jacob, R.A., D.S. Kelley, F.S. Pianalto, et al. "Immunocompetence and Oxidant Defense During Ascorbate Depletion of Healthy Men." *Am J Clin Nutr* 54:6 Suppl (1991): 1302S–1309S.

14. Hemilä, H., and Z.S. Herman. "Vitamin C and the Common Cold: A Retrospective Analysis of Chalmers' Review." *J Am Coll Nutr* 14 (1995): 116–123.

15. Douglas, R.M., H. Hemilä, R. D'Souza, et al. "Vitamin C for Preventing and Treating the Common Cold." *Cochrane Database Syst Rev* 3 (2007): CD000980.

16. Hemilä, H., and P. Louhiala. "Vitamin C for Preventing and Treating Pneumonia." *Cochrane Database Syst Rev* 1 (2007): CD005532.

17. Cathcart, R.F. "Vitamin C, Titrating to Bowel Tolerance, Anascorbemia, and Acute Induced Scurvy." *Med Hypotheses* 7 (1981): 1359–1376.

18. Ibid.

19. Shankar, A.H. "Nutritional Modulation of Immune Function and Infectious Disease." In Bowman, B.A., and R.M. Russell (eds.). *Present Knowledge in Nutrition,* 8th Edition. Washington, DC: ILSI Press, 2001, pp. 686–700.

20. Ibid.

21. Meydani, S.N., M. Meydani, J.B. Blumberg, et al. "Vitamin E Supplementation and in Vivo Immune Response in Healthy Elderly Subjects. A Randomized Controlled Trial." *JAMA* 277 (1997): 1380–1386.

22. Meydani, S.N., L.S. Leka, B.C. Fine, et al. "Vitamin E and Respiratory

Tract Infections in Elderly Nursing Home Residents: A Randomized Controlled Trial." *JAMA* 292 (2004): 828–836.

23. Ronzio, R.A. "Nutritional Support for the Immune System." *Am J Nat Med* 5:3 (1998): 18–22.

24. Grimble, R.F. "Effect of Antioxidative Vitamins on Immune Function with Clinical Applications." *Int J Vitamin Nutr Res* 67 (1997): 312–320.

25. Rall, L.C., and S.N. Meydani. "Vitamin B6 and Immune Competence." *Nutr Rev* 51 (1993): 217–225.

26. Cheng, C.H., S.J. Chang, B.J. Lee, et al. "Vitamin B6 Supplementation Increases Immune Responses in Critically Ill Patients." *Eur J Clin Nutr* 60 (2006): 1207–1213. Casciato, D.A., L.P. McAdam, J.D. Kopple, et al. "Immunologic Abnormalities in Hemodialysis Patients: Improvement after Pyridoxine Therapy." *Nephron* 38 (1984): 9–16. van Buuren, A.J., M.E. Louw, G.S. Shephard, et al. "The Effect of Pyridoxine Supplementation on Plasma Pyridoxal-5'-phosphate Levels in Children with the Nephrotic Syndrome." *Clin Nephrol* 28 (1987): 81–86.

27. Gaby, A.R. "'Safe Upper Levels for Nutritional Supplements: One Giant Step Backward." *J Orthomolecular Med* 3–4 (2003): 126–130.

28. Chaudary, A.N., A. Porter-Blake, P. Holford. "Indices of Pyridoxine Levels on Symptoms Associated with Toxicity: A Retrospective Study." *J Orthomolecular Med* 18 (2003): 65–76.

29. Calder, P.C. "Polyunsaturated Fatty Acids, Inflammation, and Immunity." *Lipids* 36 (2001): 1007–1024.

30. Puri, B.K. "Long-chain Polyunsaturated Fatty Acids and the Pathophysiology of Myalgic Encephalomyelitis (Chronic Fatigue Syndrome)." *J Clin Pathol* 60 (2007): 122–124.

31. Maes, M., I. Mihaylova, J.C. Leunis. "In Chronic Fatigue Syndrome, the Decreased Levels of Omega-3 Polyunsaturated Fatty Acids Are Related to Lowered Serum Zinc and Defects in T Cell Activation." *Neuro Endocrinol Lett* 26 (2005): 745–751.

32. Calder, P.C. "N-3 Polyunsaturated Fatty Acids, Inflammation, and Inflammatory Diseases." *Am J Clin Nutr* 83:6 Suppl (2006): 1505S–1519S.

33. Ventura, M.T., R. Crollo, E. Lasaracine, et al. "In Vitro Zinc Correction of Defective Granulocyte Chemotaxis in the Elderly." *IRCS Med Sci* 13 (1985): 535–536.

34. Prasad, A.S., S. Meftah, J. Abdallah, et al. "Serum Thymulin in Human Zinc Deficiency." *J Clin Invest* 82 (1988): 1202–1210. Beck, F.W.J., A.S. Prasad, J. Kaplan, et al. "Changes in Cytokine Production and T Cell Subpopulations in Experimentally Induced Zinc-deficient Humans." *Am J Physiol* 272 (1997): E1002–E1007.

35. Prasad, A.S. "Zinc Deficiency." *Br Med J* 326 (2003): 409–410.

36. Prasad, A.S., F.W. Beck, B. Bao, et al. "Zinc Supplementation Decreases Incidence of Infections in the Elderly: Effect of Zinc on Generation of Cytokines and Oxidative Stress." *Am J Clin Nutr* 85 (2007): 837–844.

37. Ryan-Harshman, M., and W. Aldoori. "The Relevance of Selenium to Immunity, Cancer, and Infectious/Inflammatory Diseases." *Can J Diet Pract Res* 66 (2005): 98–102.

38. Shankar, A.H. "Nutritional Modulation of Immune Function and Infectious Disease." In Bowman, B.A., and R.M. Russell (eds.). *Present Knowledge in Nutrition,* 8th Edition. Washington, DC: ILSI Press, 2001, pp. 686–700.

39. Broome, C.S., F. McArdle, J.A. Kyle, et al. "An Increase in Selenium Intake Improves Immune Function and Poliovirus Handling in Adults with Marginal Selenium Status." *Am J Clin Nutr* 80 (2004): 154–162.

40. High, K.P. "Nutritional Strategies to Boost Immunity and Prevent Infection in Elderly Individuals." *Clin Infect Dis* 33 (2001): 1892–1900.

41. Hurwitz, B.E., J.R. Klaus, M.M. Llabre, et al. "Suppression of Human Immunodeficiency Virus Type 1 Viral Load with Selenium Supplementation: A Randomized Controlled Trial." *Arch Intern Med* 167 (2007): 148–154. Kiremidjian-Schumacher, L., and M. Roy. "Effect of Selenium on the Immunocompetence of Patients with Head and Neck Cancer and on Adoptive Immunotherapy of Early and Established Lesions." *Biofactors* 14 (2001): 161–168.

42. Rayman, M.P. "The Use of High-selenium Yeast to Raise Selenium Status: How Does It Measure Up?" *Br J Nutr* 92 (2004): 557–573.

43. Ibid.

44. Bouic, P.J.D., and J.H. Lamprecht. "Plant Sterols and Sterolins: A Review of Their Immune-modulating Properties." *Altern Med Rev* 4 (1999): 170–177.

45. Ibid.

46. Kidd, P. "Th1/Th2 Balance: The Hypothesis, Its Limitations, and Implications for Health and Disease." *Altern Med Rev* 8 (2003): 223–246.

47. Visser, J.T., E.R. De Kloet, L. Nagelkerken. "Altered Glucocorticoid Regulation of the Immune Response in the Chronic Fatigue Syndrome." *Ann N Y Acad Sci* 917 (2000): 868–875.

48. Patarca, R. "Cytokines and Chronic Fatigue Syndrome." *Ann N Y Acad Sci* 933 (2001): 185–200.

49. "Monograph. Plant Sterols and Sterolins." *Altern Med Rev* 6 (2001): 203–206.

Chapter 7: Treating Mental Health Problems

1. Watanabe, N., R. Stewart, R. Jenkins, et al. "The Epidemiology of Chronic Fatigue, Physical Illness, and Symptoms of Common Mental Disorders: A

Cross-sectional Survey from the Second British National Survey of Psychiatric Morbidity." *J Psychosom Res* 64 (2008): 357–362.

2. Prousky, J. "Niacinamide's Potent Role in Alleviating Anxiety with Its Benzodiazepine-like Properties: A Case Report." *J Orthomolecular Med* 19 (2004): 104–110. Prousky, J. "Supplemental Niacinamide Mitigates Anxiety Symptoms: Report of Three Cases." *J Orthomolecular Med* 20 (2005): 167–178. Prousky, J. *Anxiety: Orthomolecular Diagnosis and Treatment.* Toronto, ON: CCNM Press, 2006.

3. Hoffer, A. "Vitamin B3 Dependent Child." *Schizophrenia* 3 (1971): 107–113. Hoffer, A. *Dr. Hoffer's ABC of Natural Nutrition for Children.* Kingston, ON: Quarry Press, 1999.

4. Werbach, M.R. "Adverse Effects of Nutritional Supplements." In *Foundations of Nutritional Medicine.* Tarzana, CA: Third Line Press, 1997, pp. 133–160.

5. Winter, S.L., and J.L. Boyer. "Hepatic Toxicity from Large Doses of Vitamin B3 (Nicotinamide)." *N Engl J Med* 289 (1973): 1180–1182.

6. Hoffer, A. "Vitamin B-3: Niacin and Its Amide." *Townsend Letter for Doctors and Patients* 147 (1995): 30–39.

7. Schilling, R.F. "Is Vitamin B12 a Tonic?" *Wis Med J* 70 (1971): 143–144.

8. Ellis, F.R., and S. Nasser. "A Pilot Study of Vitamin B12 in the Treatment of Tiredness." *Br J Nutr* 30 (1973): 277–283.

9. Hintikka, J., T. Tolmunen, A. Tanskanen, et al. "High Vitamin B12 Level and Good Treatment Outcome May Be Associated in Major Depressive Disorder." *BMC Psychiatry* 3 (2003): 17.

10. Lapp, C. "Using Vitamin B12 for the Management of CFS." *The CFIDS Chronicle* (November/December 1999): 14–16. Available online at: www.cfids.org/archives/1999/1999-6-article03.asp.

11. Wang, J.Y., J.N. Wu, T.L. Cherng, et al. "Vitamin D(3) Attenuates 6-Hydroxydopamineinduced Neurotoxicity in Rats." *Brain Res* 904 (2001): 67–75. Zehnder, D., R. Bland, M.C. Williams, et al. "Extrarenal Expression of 25-Hydroxyvitamin D(3)-1alpha-Hydroxylase." *J Clin Endocrinol Metab* 86 (2001): 888–894.

12. Vieth, R., S. Kimball, A. Hu, et al. "Randomized Comparison of the Effects of the Vitamin D3 Adequate Intake versus 100 mcg (4,000 IU) per Day on Biochemical Responses and the Wellbeing of Patients." *Nutr J* 3 (2004): 8.

13. Armstrong, D.J., G.K. Meenagh, I. Bickle, et al. "Vitamin D Deficiency Is Associated with Anxiety and Depression in Fibromyalgia." *Clin Rheumatol* 26 (2007): 551–554.

14. Bottiglieri, T., M. Laundy, R. Crellin, et al. "Homocysteine, Folate, Methylation, and Monoamine Metabolism in Depression." *J Neurol Neurosurg Psychiatry* 69 (2000): 228–232.

15. Abou-Saleh, M.T., and A. Coppen. "Folic Acid and the Treatment of Depression." *J Psychosom Res* 61 (2006): 285–287.

16. Bottiglieri, T., M. Laundy, R. Crellin, et al. "Homocysteine, Folate, Methylation, and Monoamine Metabolism in Depression." *J Neurol Neurosurg Psychiatry* 69 (2000): 228–232.

17. Lewis, S.J., D.A. Lawlor, G. Davey Smith, et al. "The Thermolabile Variant of MTHFR Is Associated with Depression in the British Women's Heart and Health Study and a Meta-analysis." *Mol Psychiatry* 11 (2006): 352–360.

18. Werbach, M.R., and J. Moss. "Depression." In *Textbook of Nutritional Medicine.* Tarzana, CA: Third Line Press, 1999, pp. 302–316.

19. Figueiredo, J.C., M.V. Grau, R.W. Haile, et al. "Folic Acid and Risk of Prostate Cancer: Results from a Randomized Clinical Trial." *J Natl Cancer Inst* 101 (2009): 432–435.

20. Rudin, D.O. "The Major Psychoses and Neuroses as Omega-3 Essential Fatty Acid Deficiency Syndrome: Substrate Pellagra." *Biol Psychiatry* 16 (1981): 837–850.

21. Ipatova, O.M., N.M. Prozorovskaia, V.S. Baranova, et al. "Biological Activity of Linseed Oil as the Source of Omega-3 Alpha-linolenic Acid." *Biomed Khim* 50 (2004): 25–43.

22. Logan, A. "Neurobehavioral Aspects of Omega-3 Fatty Acids: Possible Mechanisms and Therapeutic Value in Major Depression." *Altern Med Rev* 8 (2003): 410–425.

23. Green, P., H. Haggai, M. Assaf, et al. "Red Cell Membrane Omega-3 Fatty Acids Are Decreased in Nondepressed Patients with Social Anxiety Disorder." *Eur Neuropsychopharm* 16 (2006): 107–113.

24. Buydens-Branchey, L., and M. Branchey. "N-3 Polyunsaturated Fatty Acids Decrease Anxiety Feelings in a Population of Substance Abusers." *J Clin Psychopharmacol* 26 (2006): 661–665.

25. Logan, A. "Neurobehavioral Aspects of Omega-3 Fatty Acids: Possible Mechanisms and Therapeutic Value in Major Depression." *Altern Med Rev* 8 (2003): 410–425.

26. Ibid.

27. Rudin, D.O. "The Major Psychoses and Neuroses as Omega-3 Essential Fatty Acid Deficiency Syndrome: Substrate Pellagra." *Biol Psychiatry* 16 (1981): 837–850. Kinrys, G. "Hypomania Associated with Omega-3 Fatty Acids." *Arch Gen Psychiatry* 57 (2000): 715–716.

28. Werbach, M.R. "Adverse Effects of Nutritional Supplements." In *Foundations of Nutritional Medicine.* Tarzana, CA: Third Line Press, 1997, pp. 133–160.

29. Mitchell, W.A., Jr. *Foundations of Natural Therapeutics: Biochemical*

Apologetics of Naturopathic Medicine. Tempe, AZ: Southwest College Press, 1997, pp. 105–108.

30. Braverman, E.R., C.C. Pfeiffer, K. Blum, et al. *The Healing Nutrients Within,* 2nd Edition. New Canaan, CT: Keats Publishing, 1997, pp. 246–258, 290–303.

31. "Gamma-Aminobutyric Acid (GABA)—Monograph." *Altern Med Rev* 12 (2007): 274–279.

32. Braverman, E.R., C.C. Pfeiffer, K. Blum, et al. *The Healing Nutrients Within,* 2nd Edition. New Canaan, CT: Keats Publishing, 1997, pp. 246–258, 290–303.

33. Birdsall, T.C. "5-Hydroxytryptophan: A Clinically Effective Serotonin Precursor." *Altern Med Rev* 3 (1998): 271–280.

34. Kahn, R.S., H.G. Westenberg, W.M. Verhoeven, et al. "Effect of a Serotonin Precursor and Uptake Inhibitor in Anxiety Disorders: A Double-blind Comparison of 5-Hydroxytryptophan, Clomipramine and Placebo." *Int Clin Psychopharmacol* 2 (1987): 33–45. Schruers, K., R. van Diest, T. Overbeek, et al. "Acute L-5-Hydroxytryptophan Administration Inhibits Carbon Dioxide-induced Panic in Panic Disorder Patients." *Psychiatry Res* 113 (2002): 237–243.

35. Werbach, M.R., and J. Moss. "Anxiety." In *Textbook of Nutritional Medicine.* Tarzana, CA: Third Line Press, 1999, pp. 110–115.

36. Werbach, M.R. *Foundations of Nutritional Medicine.* Tarzana, CA: Third Line Press, 1997, pp. 141, 151–152, 188–189. Murray, M., and J. Pizzorno. *Encyclopedia of Natural Medicine,* 2nd Edition. Rocklin, CA: Prima Publishing, 1998, pp. 391–393.

37. Logan, A.C. "Letter to the Editor." *Altern Med Rev* 6 (2001): 4–6.

38. "*Rhodiola rosea.* Monograph." *Altern Med Rev* 7 (2002): 421–423.

39. Bystritsky, A., L. Kerwin, J.D. Feusner. "A Pilot Study of *Rhodiola rosea* (Rhodax) for Generalized Anxiety Disorder (GAD)." *J Altern Complement Med* 14 (2008): 175–180.

40. Bone, K. "Phytotherapy Review and Commentary—Phytotherapy for Chronic Fatigue and Fibromyalgia: Recent Developments." *Townsend Letter for Doctors and Patients* 295/296 (2008): 62–64.

41. "*Rhodiola rosea.* Monograph." *Altern Med Rev* 7 (2002): 421–423. Bone, K. "Phytotherapy Review and Commentary—Phytotherapy for Chronic Fatigue and Fibromyalgia: Recent Developments." *Townsend Letter for Doctors and Patients* 295/296 (2008): 62–64.

42. Cleare, A.J. "The Neuroendocrinology of Chronic Fatigue Syndrome." *Endocrine Rev* 24 (2007): 236–252.

43. "*Rhodiola rosea.* Monograph." *Altern Med Rev* 7 (2002): 421–423.

44. Anghelescu, I.G., R. Kohnen, A. Szegedi, et al. "Comparison of Hypericum Extract WS(r) 5570 and Paroxetine in Ongoing Treatment after Recovery from an Episode of Moderate to Severe Depression: Results from a Randomized Multicenter Study." *Pharmacopsychiatry* 39 (2006): 213–219. Kasper, S., I.G. Anghelescu, A. Szegedi, et al. "Superior Efficacy of St. John's Wort Extract WS(r) 5570 Compared to Placebo in Patients with Major Depression: A Randomized, Double-blind, Placebo-controlled, Multi-center Trial." *BMC Medicine* 4 (2006): 14.

45. Davidson, J.R., and K.M. Connor. "St. John's Wort in Generalized Anxiety Disorder: Three Case Reports." *J Clin Psychopharmacol* 21 (2001): 635–636. Kobak, K.A., L. Taylor, R. Futterer, et al. "St. John's Wort in Generalized Anxiety Disorder: Three More Case Reports." *J Clin Psychopharmacol* 23 (2003): 531–532. Taylor, L.H., and K.A. Kobak. "An Open-label Trial of St. John's Wort (*Hypericum perforatum*) in Obsessive-compulsive Disorder." *J Clin Psychiatry* 61 (2000): 575–578.

46. Volz, H.P., H. Murck, S. Kasper, et al. "St. John's Wort Extract (LI 160) in Somatoform Disorders: Results of a Placebo-controlled Trial." *Psychopharmacology* 164 (2002): 294–300. Müller, T., M. Mannel, H. Murck, et al. "Treatment of Somatoform Disorders with St. John's Wort: A Randomized, Double-blind and Placebo-controlled Trial." *Psychosom Med* 66 (2004): 538–547.

47. Wiebe, A., N. Elford, S. Dielman, et al. *Herbal-Drug Interactions.* Alberta, Canada: Mediscript Communications, 2006, pp. 64–65.

48. Woelk, H., K.H. Arnoldt, M. Kieser, et al. "*Ginkgo biloba* Special Extract EGb 761 in Generalized Anxiety Disorder and Adjustment Disorder with Anxious Mood: A Randomized, Double-blind, Placebo-controlled Trial." *J Psychiatry Res* 41 (2007): 472–480.

49. Hemmeter, U., B. Annen, R. Bischof, et al. "Polysomnographic Effects of Adjuvant *Ginkgo biloba* Therapy in Patients with Major Depression Medicated with Trimipramine." *Pharmacopsychiatry* 34 (2001): 50–59.

50. Benke, D., A. Barberis, S. Kopp, et al. "GABA A Receptors as in Vivo Substrate for the Anxiolytic Action of Valerenic Acid, a Major Constituent of Valerian Root Extracts." *Neuropharmacology* 56 (2009): 174–181.

51. Hattesohl, M., B. Feistel, H. Sievers, et al. "Extracts of *Valeriana officinalis* L. s.l. Show Anxiolytic and Antidepressant Effects but Neither Sedative nor Myorelaxant Properties." *Phytomedicine* 15 (2008): 2–15.

52. Rao, A.V., A. Bested, T. Beaulne, et al. "A Randomized, Double-blind, Placebo-controlled Pilot Study of a Probiotic in Emotional Symptoms of Chronic Fatigue Syndrome." *Gut Pathog* 1:1 (2009): 6.

53. Ibid.

Chapter 8: Alleviating Muscular Dysfunction

1. Arnold, D.I., G.K. Radda, P.J. Bore, et al. "Excessive Intracellular Acidosis of Skeletal Muscle on Exercise in a Patient with a Post-viral Exhaustion/Fatigue Syndrome." *Lancet* 1 (1984): 1367–1368.

2. Behan, P.O., W.M. Behan, E.J. Bell. "The Postviral Fatigue Syndrome—An Analysis of the Findings in 50 Cases." *J Infect* 10 (1985): 211–222.

3. Jammes, Y., J.G. Steinberg, O. Mambrini, et al. "Chronic Fatigue Syndrome: Assessment of Increased Oxidative Stress and Altered Muscle Excitability in Response to Incremental Exercise." *J Intern Med* 257 (2005): 299–310.

4. Shinchuk, L.M., and M.F. Holick. "Vitamin D and Rehabilitation: Improving Functional Outcomes." *Nutr Clin Pract* 22 (2007): 297–304. Gerwin, R.D. "A Review of Myofascial Pain and Fibromyalgia—Factors that Promote Their Persistence." *Acupunct Med* 23 (2005): 121–134.

5. McDaniel, M.A., S.F. Maier, G.O. Einstein. "Brain-specific Nutrients: A Memory Cure?" *Nutrition* 19 (2003): 957–975.

6. Rossini, M., O. Di Munno, G. Valentini, et al. "Double-blind, Multicenter Trial Comparing Acetyl-L-carnitine with Placebo in the Treatment of Fibromyalgia Patients." *Clin Exp Rheumatol* 25 (2007): 182–188.

7. Vermeulen, R.C., and H.R. Scholte. "Exploratory Open-label, Randomized Study of Acetyl- and Propionylcarnitine in Chronic Fatigue Syndrome." *Psychosom Med* 66 (2004): 276–282.

8. McCully, K.K., E. Malucelli, S. Iotti. "Increase of Free Mg^{2+} in the Skeletal Muscle of Chronic Fatigue Syndrome Patients." *Dyn Med* 5 (2006): 1.

9. Moorkens, G., Y. Manuel, B. Keenoy, et al. "Magnesium Deficit in a Sample of the Belgian Population Presenting with Chronic Fatigue." *Magnes Res* 10 (1997): 329–337.

10. Magaldi, M., L. Moltoni, G. Biasi, et al. "Changes in Intracellular Calcium and Magnesium Ions in the Physiopathology of the Fibromyalgia Syndrome." *Minerva Med* 91 (2000): 137–140.

11. Abraham, G.E., and J.D. Flechas. "Management of Fibromyalgia: Rationale for the Use of Magnesium and Malic Acid." *J Nutr Med* 3 (1991): 49–59.

12. Russell, I.J., J.E. Michalek, J.D. Flechas, et al. "Treatment of Fibromyalgia Syndrome with Super Malic: A Randomized, Double-blind, Placebo-controlled, Crossover Pilot Study." *J Rheumatol* 22 (1995): 953–958.

13. Juhl, J.H. "Fibromyalgia and the Serotonin Pathway." *Altern Med Rev* 3 (1998): 367–375.

14. Caruso, I., P. Sarzi Puttini, M. Cazzola, et al. "Double-blind Study of 5-Hydroxytryptophan versus Placebo in the Treatment of Primary Fibromyalgia Syndrome." *J Int Med Res* 18 (1990): 201–209. Sarzi Puttini, P., and I. Caru-

so. "Primary Fibromyalgia Syndrome and 5-Hydroxy-L-tryptophan: A 90-day Open Study." *J Int Med Res* 20 (1992): 182–189.

15. Goodnick, P.J., and R. Sandoval. "Psychotropic Treatment of Chronic Fatigue Syndrome and Related Disorders." *J Clin Psychiatry* 54 (1993): 13–20.

16. Werbach, M.R., and J. Moss. "Anxiety." In *Textbook of Nutritional Medicine.* Tarzana, CA: Third Line Press, 1999, pp. 110–115. Werbach, M.R. *Foundations of Nutritional Medicine.* Tarzana, CA: Third Line Press, 1997, pp. 141, 151–152, 188–189.

17. Logan, A.C. "Letter to the Editor." *Altern Med Rev* 6 (2001): 4–6.

18. Teitelbaum, J.E., C. Johnson, J. St. Cyr. "The Use of D-ribose in Chronic Fatigue Syndrome and Fibromyalgia: A Pilot Study." *J Altern Complement Med* 12 (2006): 857–862.

Chapter 9: Treating Red Blood Cell Abnormalities and Oxidative Stress

1. Simpson, L.O. "The Role of Nondiscocytic Erythrocytes in the Pathogenesis of Myalgic Encephalomyelitis/Chronic Fatigue Syndrome." In Hyde, B.M. (ed.). *Clinical and Scientific Basis of Myalgic Encephalomyelitis/Chronic Fatigue Syndrome.* Ottawa, ON, Canada: Nightingale Research Foundation, 1992, pp. 597–605.

2. Simpson, L.O., B.I. Shand, R.J. Olds. "Blood Rheology and Myalgic Encephalomyelitis: A Pilot Study." *Pathology* 18 (1986): 190–192.

3. Mukherjee, T.M., K. Smith, K. Maros. "Abnormal Red Cell Morphology in Myalgic Encephalomyelitis." *Lancet* 2 (1987): 328–329.

4. Simpson, L.O. "Nondiscocytic Erythrocytes in Myalgic Encephalomyelitis." *N Z Med J* 102 (1989): 126–127.

5. Simpson, L.O. "The Role of Nondiscocytic Erythrocytes in the Pathogenesis of Myalgic Encephalomyelitis/Chronic Fatigue Syndrome." In Hyde, B.M. (ed.). *Clinical and Scientific Basis of Myalgic Encephalomyelitis/Chronic Fatigue Syndrome.* Ottawa, ON, Canada: Nightingale Research Foundation, 1992, pp. 597–605.

6. Simpson, L.O., and G.P. Herbison. "The Results from Red Cell Shape Analyses of Blood Samples from Members of Myalgic Encephalomyelitis Organisations in Four Countries." *J Orthomolecular Med* 12 (1997): 221–226.

7. Simpson, L.O., and D.J. O'Neill. "Red Blood Cell Shape, Symptoms and Reportedly Helpful Treatments in Americans with Chronic Disorders." *J Orthomolecular Med* 16 (2001): 157–165.

8. Simpson, L.O. "The Role of Nondiscocytic Erythrocytes in the Pathogenesis of Myalgic Encephalomyelitis/Chronic Fatigue Syndrome." In Hyde, B.M. (ed.). *Clinical and Scientific Basis of Myalgic Encephalomyelitis/Chronic Fatigue Syndrome.* Ottawa, ON, Canada: Nightingale Research Foundation,

1992, pp. 597–605. Simpson, L.O. "Myalgic Encephalomyelitis (ME): A Haemorheological Disorder Manifested as Impaired Capillary Blood Flow." *J Orthomolecular Med* 12 (1997): 69–76.

9. Simpson, L.O. "Myalgic Encephalomyelitis (ME): A Haemorheological Disorder Manifested as Impaired Capillary Blood Flow." *J Orthomolecular Med* 12 (1997): 69–76.

10. Richards, R.S., T.K. Roberts, R. Hugh Dunstan, et al. "Free Radicals in Chronic Fatigue Syndrome: Cause or Effect?" *Redox Report* 5 (2000): 146–147. Richards, R.S., L. Wang, H. Jelinek. "Erythrocyte Oxidative Damage in Chronic Fatigue Syndrome." *Arch Med Res* 38 (2007): 94–98.

11. Richards, R.S., L. Wang, H. Jelinek. "Erythrocyte Oxidative Damage in Chronic Fatigue Syndrome." *Arch Med Res* 38 (2007): 94–98.

12. Pall, M.L. "Cobalamin Used in Chronic Fatigue Syndrome Therapy Is a Nitric Oxide Scavenger." *J Chronic Fatigue Syndr* 8 (2001): 39–44.

13. Simpson, L.O. "The Role of Nondiscocytic Erythrocytes in the Pathogenesis of Myalgic Encephalomyelitis/Chronic Fatigue Syndrome." In Hyde, B.M. (ed.). *Clinical and Scientific Basis of Myalgic Encephalomyelitis/Chronic Fatigue Syndrome.* Ottawa, ON, Canada: Nightingale Research Foundation, 1992, pp. 597–605.

14. Simpson, L.O. "Myalgic Encephalomyelitis (ME): A Haemorheological Disorder Manifested as Impaired Capillary Blood Flow." *J Orthomolecular Med* 12 (1997): 69–76.

15. Lapp, C. "Using Vitamin B-12 for the Management of CFS." *The CFIDS Chronicle* (November/December 1999): 14–16. Available online at: www.cfids.org/archives/1999/1999-6-article03.asp.

16. Ali, M. "Ascorbic Acid Reverses Abnormal Erythrocyte Morphology in Chronic Fatigue Syndrome." [Abstract #117.] *Am J Clin Pathol* 94 (1990): 515.

17. Shiva Shankar Reddy, C.S., M.V. Subramanyam, R. Vani, et al. "In Vitro Models of Oxidative Stress in Rat Erythrocytes: Effect of Antioxidant Supplements." *Toxicol In Vitro* 21 (2007): 1355–1364. Traber, M.G., B. Frei, J.S. Beckman. "Vitamin E Revisited: Do New Data Validate Benefits for Chronic Disease Prevention?" *Curr Opin Lipidol* 19 (2008): 30–38.

18. Simpson, L.O. "Myalgic Encephalomyelitis (ME): A Haemorheological Disorder Manifested as Impaired Capillary Blood Flow." *J Orthomolecular Med* 12 (1997): 69–76.

19. Puri, B.K. "Long-chain Polyunsaturated Fatty Acids and the Pathophysiology of Myalgic Encephalomyelitis (Chronic Fatigue Syndrome)." *J Clin Pathol* 60 (2007): 122–124.

20. Simpson, L.O. "Myalgic Encephalomyelitis (ME): A Haemorheological Disorder Manifested as Impaired Capillary Blood Flow." *J Orthomolecular Med* 12 (1997): 69–76.

21. Manku, M.S., D.F. Horrobin, N. Morse, et al. "Reduced Levels of Prostaglandin Precursors in the Blood of Atopic Patients: Defective Delta-6-desaturase Function as a Biochemical Basis for Atopy." *Prostaglandins Leukot Med* 9 (1982): 615–628.

22. Maes, M., I. Mihaylova, J.C. Leunis. "In Chronic Fatigue Syndrome, the Decreased Levels of Omega-3 Poly-unsaturated Fatty Acids Are Related to Lowered Serum Zinc and Defects in T Cell Activation." *Neuro Endocrinol Lett* 26 (2005): 745–751.

23. Fischler, L., D.O. Meredith, W.H. Reinhart. "Influence of a Parenteral Fish-oil Preparation (Omegaven) on Erythrocyte Morphology and Blood Viscosity in Vitro." *Clin Hemorheol Microcirc* 28 (2003): 79–88.

24. Simpson, L.O., E.G. McQueen, B.I. Shand, et al. "Changes in Red Cell Shape in Healthy Elderly Subjects Taking Low-dose Fish Oil: Pilot Study." *N Z Med J* 104 (1991): 316–318.

25. Bested, A.C., P.R. Saunders, A.C. Logan. "Chronic Fatigue Syndrome: Neurological Findings May Be Related to Blood-Brain Barrier Permeability." *Med Hypotheses* 57 (2001): 231–237.

26. Rosenblat, M., N. Volkova, R. Coleman, et al. "Anti-oxidant and Anti-atherogenic Properties of Liposomal Glutathione: Studies in Vitro, and in the Atherosclerotic Apolipoprotein E-deficient Mice." *Atherosclerosis* 195 (2007): 61–68.

27. Logan, A.C., and C. Wong. "Chronic Fatigue Syndrome: Oxidative Stress and Dietary Modifications." *Altern Med Rev* 6 (2001): 450–459.

28. Feher, G., K. Koltai, G. Kesmarky, et al. "Effect of Parenteral or Oral Vinpocetine on the Hemorheological Parameters of Patients with Chronic Cerebrovascular Diseases." *Phytomedicine* 16 (2009): 111–117.

29. Rasmussen, H., W. Lake, J.E. Allen. "The Effect of Catecholamines and Prostaglandins upon Human and Rat Erythrocytes." *Biochim Biophys Acta* 411 (1975): 63–73. Ehrly, A.M., H. Landgraf, J. Hessler, et al. "Influence of Video Film-induced Emotional Stress on the Flow Properties of Blood." *Angiology* 39 (1988): 341–344.

30. Logan, A.C. "Letter to the Editor." *Altern Med Rev* 6 (2001): 4–6.

31. A more detailed description of this case appeared in: Prousky, J. *Principles and Practices of Naturopathic Clinical Nutrition*. Toronto, ON: CCNM Press, pp. 225–226.

INDEX

About the Author

Jonathan E. Prousky graduated from Bastyr University (Kenmore, WA) with a doctorate in Naturopathic Medicine and completed a Family Practice Residency sponsored by the National College of Naturopathic Medicine (now known as National College of Natural Medicine). As the Chief Naturopathic Medical Officer at the Canadian College of Naturopathic Medicine, Dr. Prousky's primary responsibility is the delivery of safe, effective naturopathic medical care. His private practice focus is on optimizing mental and neurological health with nutrition and botanical medicines. He has lectured extensively on various health-related topics throughout North America to medical doctors, naturopathic doctors, other health-care providers, and laypeople. Dr. Prousky is the author of *Anxiety: Orthomolecular Diagnosis and Treatment*, *Naturopathic Nutrition* (with Abram Hoffer, Ph.D., M.D.) and *Principles and Practices of Naturopathic Clinical Nutrition*.